Diabetes Nutrition A to Z

What You Need to Know About Diabetes Nutrition–Simply Put

Follows the ADA Nutrition Recommendations for 2001

Lea Ann Holzmeister, RD, CDE
Patti B. Geil, MS, RD, FADA, CDE

American Diabetes Association®
Cure • Care • Commitment℠

Director, Book Publishing, John Fedor; *Associate Director*, *Consumer Books*, Sherrye Landrum; *Editor*, Laurie Guffey; *Production Manager*, Peggy M. Rote; *Composition*, Circle Graphics, Inc.; *Cover Design*, Wickham & Associates, Inc.; *Printer*, XXXXXXXXXXXX.

Printed in the United States of America
1 3 5 7 9 10 8 6 4 2

The suggestions and information contained in this publication are generally consistent with the *Clinical Practice Recommendations* and other policies of the American Diabetes Association, but they do not represent the policy or position of the Association or any of its boards or committees. Reasonable steps have been taken to ensure the accuracy of the information presented. However, the American Diabetes Association cannot ensure the safety or efficacy of any product or service described in this publication. Individuals are advised to consult a physician or other appropriate health care professional before undertaking any diet or exercise program or taking any medication referred to in this publication. Professionals must use and apply their own professional judgment, experience, and training and should not rely solely on the information contained in this publication before prescribing any diet, exercise, or medication. The American Diabetes Association—its officers, directors, employees, volunteers, and members—assumes no responsibility or liability for personal or other injury, loss, or damage that may result from the suggestions or information in this publication.

The paper in this publication meets the requirements of the ANSI Standard Z39.48-1992 ♾ (permanence of paper).

ADA titles may be purchased for business or promotional use or for special sales. For information, please write to Lee Romano Sequeira, Special Sales & Promotions, at the address below.

American Diabetes Association
1701 North Beauregard Street
Alexandria, Virginia 22311

Library of Congress Cataloging-in-Publication Data
Holzmeister, Lea Ann.
Diabetes nutrition A to Z / Lea Ann Holzmeister, Patti Bazel Geil.
p. cm.
Includes index.
ISBN 1-58040-051-5
1. Diabetes—Nutritional aspects—Encyclopedias. I. Geil, Patti Bazel. II. Title.

RC622 .H663 2001
616.4'620654'03—dc21

2001041328

A special thanks to:

Jack, Kristen, and Rachel
Jeff, Erin, Adam, and Emily

We appreciate your support through all it took for us to put this book together, from **A**uthors' block to lack of **Z**zz's and everything in between!

PBG
LAH

Contents

1 Adolescence
3 Alcohol
5 American Association of Diabetes Educators
6 American Diabetes Association
7 American Dietetic Association
8 Antioxidants
10 Appetite Suppressants (Diet Pills)
12 Athletes
14 Behavior Change
16 Blood Fats (Lipids)
20 Blood Glucose
22 Blood Glucose Monitoring
25 Breastfeeding
27 Caffeine
29 Calories
31 Carbohydrate
34 Carbohydrate Counting
37 Carbohydrate Loading
39 Carbohydrate-to-Insulin Ratio
41 Celiac Disease
43 Certified Diabetes Educator (CDE)
45 Children (Ages 6–11)
47 Cholesterol (Dietary)
49 Complications

52 Constipation
54 Convenience Foods
56 Conventional Therapy
58 Cow's Milk
60 DASH Diet
62 Dehydration/Fluid Requirements
64 Diabetes Control and Complications Trial (DCCT)
66 Diabetes Food Pyramid
69 Dietary Guidelines for Americans
71 Dietary Reference Intakes (DRIs)
73 Diverticulosis
75 Eating Disorders
78 Eggs
80 Elderly
82 Electrolytes
84 Ethnic Foods
86 *Exchange Lists for Meal Planning*
88 Exercise (Physical Activity)
93 Fast Food
95 Fat Replacers
97 Fats and Oils
101 Fiber
103 *First Step in Diabetes Meal Planning*
105 Food Diaries
107 Food Labels
109 Food Safety
111 Free Foods
113 Fructosamine Test
115 Gestational Diabetes Mellitus (GDM)
118 Glucagon
120 Glucose Intolerance
122 Glycemic Index
124 Glycohemoglobin Test

126 Goal Setting
128 Gram
129 Grocery Shopping
131 *Healthy Food Choices*
133 Heart Disease
136 Herbals and Supplements
139 Honeymoon Phase
141 Hyperglycemia
144 Hypertension
146 Hypoglycemia
149 Insulin
152 Insulin Pump Therapy
154 Intensive Insulin Therapy
157 Internet Nutrition Advice
159 Ketones
161 Kidney Disease
164 Legumes
166 Low-Carbohydrate Diets
168 Meal Planning
170 Medical Foods
171 Medical Nutrition Therapy
172 Metabolism
174 National Diabetes Education Program (NDEP)
175 "New Wave" Nutrition Definitions
178 Nutrition Recommendations for People with Diabetes
181 Obesity
183 Oral Diabetes Medicines
186 Osteoporosis
189 Percent Daily Values
191 Point or Counting Systems
194 Portion Control
196 Pregnancy
200 Preventing Diabetes

203 Protein
205 Recipes
207 Registered Dietitian
209 Resistant Starch
210 Restaurant Dining
212 Sick Days
214 Snacks
216 Sodium
218 Soy
220 Special Occasions
222 Sugar Alcohols
224 Sugar Substitutes
226 Sugars and Sweets
228 Toddlers
230 Total Available Glucose
231 Travel
234 Type 1 Diabetes
236 Type 2 Diabetes
238 Type 2 Diabetes in Youth
240 United Kingdom Prospective Diabetes Study (UKPDS)
242 Vegetarian Diets
245 Vitamins and Minerals
248 Weight Control
251 Whole Grains
253 Index

Adolescence

By adolescence, many teenagers are major decision-makers in their food choices and their diabetes management. Just when a teen is primed to take on some of the diabetes management tasks, phenomenal growth and raging hormones can strike a huge blow to diabetes control. Glucose control gets harder and harder to achieve as the need for insulin increases. Parents must balance the need to stay involved without being overbearing. Gradually shifting diabetes management from parent to teen, with parents continuing to participate in a supportive way, helps maintain sanity and blood glucose control.

Parents have far less control over what their teenager eats, but they continue to take the responsibility of having foods available for meals and snacks. Teenagers influence family eating by sharing food shopping and preparation. It is also likely that they eat more food and beverages away from home, especially fast food. Laying the groundwork for the basics of nutrition and healthy eating during the early childhood influences teen choices. However, peer pressure, school and work schedules, a sense of independence, lack of personal discipline, and unrealistic notions about body weight can get in the way of healthy eating.

Teens benefit from knowing how to make food choices to help control their diabetes, rather than letting their diabetes control them. Teens can learn how to think ahead and plan how to manage parties, sports events, late night snacks, sleeping late, and fast food. To problem-solve these situations, teens can think about options. There may be a need for a change in the food plan, exercise plan, insulin quantity and type, or schedule. Teens may benefit from the tools of intensive therapy, multiple injections, or insulin pumps, as well as insulin adjustments for changes in food and activity. The next step in problem solving is monitoring and evaluating the results of changes. These basic problem-solving steps give teens flexibility and freedom.

Useful References

- **Web Sites**

  www.childrenwithdiabetes.com
  www.jdfcure.org

- **Books**

  Sweet Kids: How to Balance Diabetes Control & Good Nutrition with Family Peace by Betty Brackenridge and Richard Rubin. Published by the American Diabetes Association, 1996.

  In Control—A Guide for Teens with Diabetes by Jean Betschart and Susan Thom. Published by John Wiley & Sons, Inc., 1995.

  Getting a Grip on Diabetes: Quick Tips & Techniques for Kids and Teens by Spike and Bo Nasmyth Loy. Published by the American Diabetes Association, 2001.

Alcohol

The Dietary Guidelines for Americans state, "If you drink alcoholic beverages, do so in moderation." For people with diabetes, this same precaution applies. It is important, however, to avoid alcohol if your blood glucose is too high or too low, if you have a history of alcohol abuse, if you are pregnant, or if you have other medical problems such as neuropathy, pancreatitis, and very high triglyceride levels. Some medications, including diabetes medications, require limits on alcohol use. Alcohol may interact with medicine, either making it less effective or more potent. Excessive alcohol intake (three or more drinks per day) is a risk factor for hypertension and stroke. However, light to moderate alcohol intake may actually be associated with a reduced risk of type 2 diabetes, coronary heart disease and stroke.

Moderate drinking is defined as no more than one drink a day for women and two drinks a day for men. Women absorb alcohol more efficiently than men do and they also weigh less, making them more susceptible to the effects of alcohol. One drink is 12 ounces of beer, 5 ounces of wine, or 1 1/2 ounces of 80-proof distilled spirits.

Alcohol can make blood glucose too high or too low. If you drink alcohol without eating food and you take diabetes pills or insulin, your blood glucose may go too low. This happens because alcohol, a toxin, is in the body and the liver attempts to get rid of it first. While the liver is busy breaking down the alcohol, it cannot release glucose into your blood and your blood glucose may go too low. When used in moderation and with food, blood glucose levels are not affected by the ingestion of alcohol. To avoid low blood glucose, eat something when you drink alcohol and check your blood glucose before, during, and after prolonged drinking. Alcohol can lower your blood glucose level from 6 to 36 hours afterwards.

Signs of too much alcohol, such as slurred speech and confusion, are similar to low blood glucose signs and symptoms. If you have low blood glucose while drinking, it is important to let others know that you have diabetes and are not drunk. Wear a medical identification bracelet in case you are unable to talk.

The alcohol and sugars in many drinks give you calories and can cause blood glucose levels to go too high. Choose lower calorie mixers such as mineral water, club soda, diet tonic water, diet soda, coffee, or tomato juice. Choose light beer or a glass of wine. If you have type 2 diabetes or are overweight, check with your registered dietitian for help.

Drink	Serving (oz)	Calories	Carbohydrate (g)
Light beer	12	100	5
Regular beer	12	150	13
Nonalcoholic beer	12	60	12
Dry wine	4	80–85	0–2
Sweet wine	4	105	5
Wine cooler	12	215	30
Liquor	1.5	107	0

American Association of Diabetes Educators

The American Association of Diabetes Educators (AADE) is a multidisciplinary organization representing more than 10,000 health care professionals who provide diabetes education and care. Diabetes educators are nurses, dietitians, pharmacists, exercise specialists, physicians, and social workers who work in a variety of settings ranging from private offices to nursing homes to clinics. Certified diabetes educators (CDEs) have met education and practice requirements as well as passed a certification examination, all designed to promote excellence in the profession of diabetes education. See page 43 for more information about Certified Diabetes Educators.

A diabetes educator can create an individual self-management plan that promotes independence and good health. You can find a diabetes educator through AADE's web site at www.aadenet.org. The headquarters of the American Association of Diabetes Educators is in Chicago and can be reached at 800-832-6874.

American Diabetes Association

The American Diabetes Association (ADA) is the nation's leading nonprofit health organization providing diabetes research, information, and advocacy. The mission of the ADA is to prevent and cure diabetes and to improve the lives of all people affected by diabetes. The organization does this by supporting research; providing information and services to people with diabetes, their families, health care professionals, and the public; as well as promoting legislation and advocating for the rights of people with diabetes.

The ADA provides a wealth of information about diabetes nutrition via their web site at www.diabetes.org. To find a diabetes education program that is an American Diabetes Association Recognized Diabetes Education Program, call 800-232-0822. The headquarters of the American Diabetes Association is in Alexandria, Va., and can be reached at 800-342-2383.

American Dietetic Association

The American Dietetic Association (ADA), with nearly 70,000 members, is the largest organization of food and nutrition professionals in the nation. The mission of ADA is to serve the public through the promotion of optimal nutrition, health, and well being.

Approximately 75% of ADA members are registered dietitians (RDs), many of whom have special interest and training in the nutrition management of diabetes. You can find a dietitian through ADA's Nationwide Nutrition Network via their web site at www.eatright.org. The headquarters of The American Dietetic Association is in Chicago and can be reached at 800-877-1600.

Antioxidants

Antioxidants such as Vitamins A, beta-carotene (which forms Vitamin A), C, E, and selenium are being touted in the marketplace as "magic bullets" in the prevention of heart disease, cancer, and the effects of aging. Should you supplement your diet with antioxidant pills? Before you decide, it may help to know how antioxidants work. Every cell in our body needs oxygen to generate energy. In the process of using oxygen, byproducts called free radicals are formed. Free radicals are harmful compounds that can increase the potential for damage to cells throughout the body by disrupting our natural cancer-fighting defenses, destroying cell membranes, and causing more plaque to develop on blood vessel walls, contributing to the risk of heart disease. High blood glucose encourages free radicals to form in the body, where they may be involved in the development of diabetes complications.

The interest in antioxidants for diabetes began when scientists noted that individuals who ate large amounts of fruits and vegetables had lower rates of certain cancers and heart disease. Because this effect was felt to be due to antioxidants, studies were designed to investigate the effect of antioxidant pills as dietary supplements. Unfortunately, these large well-controlled studies have failed to show a beneficial effect from supplements. There may be substances in fruits and vegetables yet to be identified that play a role in the prevention of cancer and heart disease. It may be that the studies didn't last long enough to show the effects or didn't test the correct combination of antioxidants, so further research is necessary in this area.

Until the final results are in, you should know that large doses of antioxidants do not conclusively protect against heart disease, diabetes, and various forms of cancer; in fact, they may even have dangerous side effects such as bleeding, diarrhea, and other toxic reactions. The best approach is to enjoy lots of antioxidant-rich foods such as fruits and vegetables, lean protein, and healthy fats in your meal plan. The following is a list of rich sources of selected antioxidants.

- **Vitamin A and beta-carotene:** green leafy vegetables (broccoli, collard greens, kale, and spinach) and red, orange, and yellow fruits and vegetables (apricot, cantaloupe, carrot, mango, peach, pumpkin, sweet potato, tomato, watermelon, and squash).
- **Vitamin C:** broccoli, cantaloupe, citrus fruit (orange, grapefruit, lemon), guava, kiwi, papaya, potato, red pepper, strawberries, and tomato.
- **Vitamin E:** almonds, nuts, seeds, vegetable oil, and wheat germ.
- **Selenium:** cashews, halibut, meat, oysters, salmon, scallops, and tuna.

Appetite Suppressants (Diet Pills)

The medications most often used in the management of obesity are commonly known as "appetite suppressant" medications or diet pills. Weight loss drugs must be combined with physical activity and improved eating habits to lose and maintain weight successfully. They are not a substitute for adopting healthy eating habits over the long term. They have side effects and should never be taken for very long and only under your health care provider's advice.

Prescription appetite suppressants promote weight loss by decreasing appetite, increasing the feeling of being full, or decreasing the absorption of fat. Medications that decrease appetite act by increasing serotonin or catecholamine—two brain chemicals that affect mood and appetite. These diet drugs cause you to feel less hungry, making it easier to stick to a low-calorie diet. These medications may cause symptoms of sleeplessness, nervousness, euphoria (feeling of well being) and elevations in blood pressure and heart rate. Medications that decrease the absorption of fat in the intestine are called lipase inhibitors. They work by reducing the amount of fat that can be absorbed during digestion by about 30%. The fat is lost in the stools, leading to side effects of oily or loose stools and intestinal gas.

Many over-the-counter diet pills claiming to help with weight loss are also available. Most of these medications act as stimulants and decrease appetite. The safety and effectiveness of over-the-counter weight loss drugs have not been determined. Herbal preparations for weight loss are seldom labeled with amounts of active ingredients, so knowing how much of a drug you're getting is nearly impossible. Some have unpleasant side effects and some can be addictive or dangerous, with potential damage to the heart and nervous system.

If you and your health care provider believe that appetite suppressants may be helpful for you, it is important to discuss the goals of treatment. Improving your health and reducing your diabetes risk should be the primary goals. A modest weight loss of 5 to 10% of your starting weight can improve your health. Find out what type of program will be provided along with the medication to help you improve your eating and physical activity habits. Your response to the medication—not only in terms of weight loss, but how it affects your overall health—should be monitored regularly by your health care provider.

Useful Reference

- **Web Site**
  www.niddk.nih.gov/health/nutrit/win.htm

Athletes

Exercise may be a way of life for the elite professional athlete, or it may be an organized activity for the student athlete. For the athlete with diabetes, proper planning and advances in blood glucose monitoring technology offer a safe approach for balancing insulin and energy needs. Good nutrition and adequate energy play an important role in the regulation of blood glucose levels before, during, and after physical activities. Taking in an adequate supply of fluids and fuel are important to prevent fatigue and ensure peak athletic performance.

Each athlete has an individual metabolic response to exercise. Insulin requirements decrease as the intensity and duration of exercise increases. For the elite athlete, insulin dosage is often decreased in anticipation of intense exercise. Energy (calorie) requirements are higher for athletes. In general, exercisers take approximately 60% of their total energy requirements from carbohydrate. The goal, however, in determining a food plan and insulin requirements is to maintain blood glucose control and prevent glycosuria. Calorie and carbohydrate requirements can be determined from a detailed nutrition history and the help of your registered dietitian.

Although all athletes will eventually need fuel replacements during exercise, individuals with diabetes may need replenishment of fuel, especially carbohydrates, sooner. Blood glucose levels may drop sooner, faster, and to lower levels in the exerciser with diabetes. Athletes with diabetes should eat 15 grams of carbohydrate before or after exercise lasting one hour or less. For every hour during a long event, athletes should take in 10–15 grams of carbohydrate. For very intense or competitive activities, such as a marathon, athletes may need 10–15 grams of carbohydrate every 30 minutes. Fluid sources of carbohydrate are recommended for exercise lasting longer than 60 minutes. (See page 89–91 for more specific information on replenishment of fuel for exercise.)

Athletes with diabetes vary in their response to training and physical stress. Adjustments that work for one person may not work for another. It is important to keep training logs of the type, duration, and the intensity of exercise as well as records of blood glucose monitoring, food ingestion, insulin dose, and site of injection. This data helps you and your health care professionals identify patterns and plan a safe exercise-training schedule.

Useful References

Web Sites

www.diabetes-exercise.org

www.acsm.org

Books

The "I Hate to Exercise" Book for People with Diabetes by Charlotte Hayes. Published by the American Diabetes Association, 2000.

Safe and Healthy Exercise (booklet). Published by the International Diabetes Center, 1999.

The Fitness Book for People with Diabetes. Published by the American Diabetes Association, 1994.

Behavior Change

Planning nutritious meals is one of the most challenging aspects of living with diabetes. For people with diabetes to follow a healthy meal plan, it takes more than knowledge about the importance of nutrition. Other factors such as motivation, resources, and support from family are involved in making a behavioral change. Making changes in any aspect of your lifestyle often involves a process or series of behavior changes as outlined by a researcher named Prochaska. The five stages in the process of changing a specific behavior are listed below.

- **Pre-contemplation:** not considering a change, do not even consciously recognize there is a real need to change.
- **Contemplation:** aware that a problem exists, thinking about making a change.
- **Preparation:** decided to change, actively planning how to accomplish the change.
- **Action:** implementing the plan to make changes.
- **Maintenance:** continuing new behaviors and working to prevent relapse.

Progression through the stages of change is not linear, because you may relapse and recycle back through earlier stages. You may cycle through the stages several times before you succeed in you effort to change behavior. For example, you may implement a goal of measuring your food at meals to decrease portion sizes and calorie intake. After ten days of measuring your food, you find yourself relapsing to only measuring at breakfast. Then it would be important to evaluate your decision to make a change and re-plan how to accomplish the change.

Diabetes is primarily a self-managed disease, where you are in charge of and responsible for your care. Decisions about making changes in your lifestyle are yours. However, your health care provider is available to help guide you through changing lifestyle behaviors. It is important for you and them to identify your readiness to make changes before specific interventions are suggested. Consider your readiness to make changes in your life at a particular time and communicate this to your health care professional. Your awareness of the behavior change process will make your consultations efficient and successful.

Useful References

- **Web Sites**

  www.diabetes.org
  www.diabetes123.com

- **Books**

  When Diabetes Hits Home: The Whole Family's Guide to Finding Emotional Health by Wendy Satin Rapaport. Published by the American Diabetes Association, 1998.

  Caring for the Diabetic Soul: Successful Strategies for Coping with the Emotional Stress of Diabetes. Published by the American Diabetes Association, 1997.

Blood Fats (Lipids)

Fats are part of every cell in your body, where they perform a full range of functions. Fats work as a partner in your body, supporting the work of other nutrients. Fat supplies energy, or calories, to power physical activity. They are part of hormones and provide a protective coating to nerve cells and organs. Extra fat is stored in your body's fatty tissues, mostly in fat cells. Cholesterol and triglycerides are two blood fats made by the body that can affect your risk for heart disease. You can also get these fats from the animal foods you eat.

Cholesterol and triglycerides are carried through your blood in protein-coated packages called lipoproteins. Without the protein coating, lipids or fat cannot travel through the blood stream. Three kinds of lipoproteins are listed below.

- **Very-low-density lipoproteins (VLDLs):** VLDLs carry triglycerides, cholesterol, and other fats from the liver to other parts of the body. As VLDLs travel through your bloodstream, they lose triglycerides, pick up cholesterol, and turn into low-density lipoproteins.

- **Low-density lipoproteins (LDLs):** LDLs, sometimes called "bad" cholesterol, carry cholesterol to body tissues and may form deposits (plaques) on the walls of arteries and other blood vessels. These plaques can eventually block an artery, keep blood from flowing through, and trigger a heart attack or stroke.
- **High-density lipoproteins (HDLs):** HDLs are protein and fat particles too dense and compact to pass through blood vessel walls. They carry cholesterol to the liver where it is broken down and sent out of the body. HDLs, sometimes called "good" cholesterol, can reduce the risk of heart attack.

People with diabetes, especially people with type 2 diabetes, often have abnormal blood fat levels. This may be related to obesity or diabetes. In either case, abnormal blood lipid levels can increase your risk of heart disease, heart attack, or stroke.

The ADA recommends that people with diabetes have blood lipids checked every year. Ask your health care professionals what your blood fat levels are each time you have a lipid profile. Find out how you can improve your lipid levels to decrease your health risk.

BLOOD LIPID GOALS FOR PEOPLE WITH DIABETES

Total Cholesterol	<200 mg/dl
LDL (bad) Cholesterol	<100 mg/dl
HDL (good) Cholesterol	>45 mg/dl (men) and >55 mg/dl (women)
Triglycerides	<200 mg/dl

To increase HDL cholesterol and lower LDL cholesterol and triglyceride levels:

- Improve blood glucose control. This may decrease LDL cholesterol by up to 10–15%. Losing weight can also boost your HDL cholesterol. You must improve blood glucose before other strategies will work.

- Lose weight. Even a modest weight loss will improve your blood glucose and lipids.
- Stay physically active. Exercise lowers HDL levels, reduces blood pressure, helps control stress, helps control body weight, gives your heart muscle a good workout, and improves blood glucose control.
- Stop smoking. Smoking lowers your HDL cholesterol and is a key factor in sudden death from cardiovascular disease.
- Reduce the fat in your diet to help with weight control.
- Reduce your intake of cholesterol to less than 300 milligrams per day. Some individuals may benefit from lowering dietary cholesterol to less than 200 mg per day. Choose lean meats and low-fat dairy products. Eat eggs and organ meats in moderation.
- Reduce saturated fat and trans fatty acids to no more than 10% of your calories. Some individuals may benefit from lowering saturated fat intake to less than 7% of total energy. Saturated fats are found in red meats, poultry, seafood, whole milk, cheese, butter, solid margarine, and convenience foods. Replace saturated fats or trans fatty acids with monounsaturated fats (olive oil, peanut oil, canola oil, olives, and avocados).
- Eat high-fiber foods, such as beans, oat bran, oatmeal, wheat bran, barley, and some fruits and vegetables. Soluble fiber may help lower blood cholesterol in some people.

Useful References

Web Sites

www.diabetes.org
www.americanheart.org
www.nhlbi.nih.gov

Books

The Diabetes Problem Solver: Quick Answers to Your Questions about Treatment and Self-Care by Nancy Touchette. Published by the American Diabetes Association, 1999.

The Uncomplicated Guide to Diabetes Complications by Marvin E. Levin and Michael A. Pfeifer. Published by the American Diabetes Association, 1998.

Blood Glucose

Diabetes is actually several different types of diseases with one thing in common—elevated blood glucose levels. Blood glucose (or blood sugar) is the source of energy for the cells in the body and comes from the breakdown of the foods you eat as well as the glucose made in your liver. The amount of glucose in the blood is known as the blood glucose level. Insulin is needed for the glucose from food to reach your cells to be used for energy to keep you alive. Whether you have type 1, type 2, or gestational diabetes, your insulin is either unavailable or is unable to work effectively. Because the glucose can't reach the cells, it builds up to high levels in the blood, causing the symptoms of uncontrolled diabetes. (See page 172 for more information about the metabolism of food and its relationship to diabetes.)

Too much glucose in the blood is called **hyperglycemia**, a condition in which blood glucose levels are 140 mg/dl or above. If your blood glucose is too high, you may experience symptoms such as frequent urination, increased hunger and thirst, and weight loss. Hyperglycemia can damage your body, so it's important to see your diabetes team if your blood glucose is high. (See page 141 for more information.)

If your blood glucose drops too low (generally below 70 mg/dl), you may experience **hypoglycemia**, also known as an insulin reaction. Symptoms of hypoglycemia include shakiness, confusion, sweatiness, and irritability. Hypoglycemia is a medical emergency, which if left untreated can become severe and lead to loss of consciousness. (See page 146 for more information.)

Keeping blood glucose levels within a healthy range requires a balancing act if you have diabetes. Monitoring your blood glucose levels (see page 22), taking medication if necessary, including physical activity in your lifestyle, and following an individualized meal plan will help you stay healthy and keep your blood glucose level in the target range suggested by your diabetes team.

Useful References

- **Web Sites**

  www.diabetes.org
  www.niddk.nih.gov

- **Books**

  American Diabetes Association Complete Guide to Diabetes, 2nd Edition. Published by The American Diabetes Association, 1999.

  Diabetes A to Z, 4th Edition. Published by the American Diabetes Association, 2000.

Blood Glucose Monitoring

Monitoring your blood glucose goes hand in hand with your diabetes meal plan, medication, and physical activity as you strive for improved diabetes control. You can't manage what you don't measure! Your blood glucose monitoring results are more than just numbers. With the help of your diabetes team, you will be able to discover the story behind the numbers and use this information to make changes for better glucose control.

Blood glucose monitoring is important whether you have type 1, type 2, or gestational diabetes. The number of times you monitor your blood glucose each day depends on your overall goals and the type of diabetes you have. For most people with type 1 diabetes, blood glucose should be monitored three or more times each day (before each meal and at bedtime). Some individuals with type 1 diabetes check up to seven times each day (before and after breakfast, before and after lunch, before and after dinner and at bedtime), particularly if they are newly diagnosed or using an insulin pump. If necessary, an additional test in the middle of the night (2 to 4 a.m.) may be needed. Pregnant women with diabetes may monitor their blood glucose before and after each meal as well.

If you have type 2 diabetes and are taking an oral diabetes medication or managing your diabetes with diet alone, you may not need to check as frequently. Most clinicians suggest testing at least once a day at random times to give a 24-hour profile of blood glucose levels. People with type 2 diabetes who are taking insulin should monitor their blood glucose at least twice a day. The role of blood glucose measurements taken after meals (postprandially) is becoming more important. No matter what your blood glucose monitoring schedule, you may need to check more frequently if your schedule changes, you have a change in physical activity level, an illness occurs, or if you have a change in medication or diet.

Keeping blood glucose levels as near normal as possible lowers the risk of diabetes complications. Speak with your physician and diabetes team to determine your blood glucose management goals. The American Diabetes Association supports the blood glucose goals below.

BLOOD GLUCOSE GOALS

Whole Blood Values	Normal (mg/dl)	Goal (mg/dl)	Take Action If Glucose Is:
Premeal	<100	80–120	<80 or >140
Bedtime	<110	100–140	<100 or >160
Plasma Values	**Normal (mg/dl)**	**Goal (mg/dl)**	**Take Action**
Premeal	<110	90–130	<90 or >150
Bedtime	<120	110–150	<110 or >180

Because many laboratories measure plasma glucose levels, you'll find that most newer home blood glucose monitors now calibrate whole blood values to plasma values. Plasma glucose values are 10–15% higher than whole blood values, so it is crucial that you know which type of information your monitor and strips provide.

Keep a record of your blood glucose monitoring results and look for patterns in the values. Finding a pattern will document problems and enable you to develop a plan of action. For example, you may find you tend to have low blood glucose an hour before lunch. Possible solutions to the problem include adjusting the time, type, or dose of your morning medication; adding a midmorning snack; or increasing the amount of food in your breakfast. You may also be able to figure out the reason behind an unexpectedly high or low level. It could be related to eating too much food, but high levels can also be due to stress, illness, infection, change in physical activity, or incorrect medication dosage. Knowing your blood glucose numbers can help you make the changes you need to achieve good diabetes control.

Useful Reference

- **Book**

  American Diabetes Association Complete Guide to Diabetes, 2nd Edition. Published by the American Diabetes Association, 1999.

Breastfeeding

Breast milk is the best source of nutrition for your baby and it offers many physical, emotional, and practical benefits. Breastfeeding is recommended for women with diabetes, though it can complicate blood glucose control. Discuss your plans to breastfeed with your diabetes health care professionals before you deliver. Ask for help in identifying your blood glucose goals and your meal plan for breastfeeding.

The extra energy your body uses to make breast milk lowers blood glucose and requires an extra 500 calories a day. Your meal plan during pregnancy may meet your needs initially after delivery, but your appetite and calorie needs may increase as your baby's demand for milk increases. You may gradually lose one to two pounds per month. Develop a breastfeeding meal plan with your registered dietitian. Breastfeeding mothers may require less insulin because of the calories expended with nursing. The intermediate-acting insulin may be given at bedtime, because of the risk for hypoglycemia following nighttime breastfeeding. You must monitor your blood glucose carefully to adjust your insulin to your new eating and sleeping patterns and your infant's demands for milk. Checking your blood glucose right before nursing is wise.

Since breastfeeding lowers blood glucose levels, eat a snack such as a glass of milk, piece of fruit, or a small bowl of cereal before or during breastfeeding. It helps to have your snack or meal portion ready to eat when your baby is ready to nurse. Snacking or eating while your infant nurses helps prevent low blood glucose and replenishes fluids and energy. Eating a meal 1–2 hours before nursing works well also. Try to nap after meals or snacks and not before, because you may sleep through your eating time and cause low blood glucose. During nighttime feedings, have a snack yourself to help prevent hypoglycemia, especially in the early morning.

Women with diabetes can breastfeed successfully, but the decision to breastfeed or use commercial infant formula is a personal one. Discuss questions or concerns with your diabetes professionals and your pediatrician.

Useful Reference

- **Book**
  Diabetes and Pregnancy: What to Expect, 4th Edition. Published by the American Diabetes Association, 2001.

Caffeine

Caffeine is a mild stimulant found naturally occurring in plants. We consume caffeine in products such as coffee, chocolate, tea, and cola drinks. Caffeine is also used as an ingredient in more than 1000 over-the-counter drugs and prescription drugs.

Over the years, studies have explored the connection between caffeine and diabetes. One study reported enhanced warning symptoms or ability to recognize hypoglycemia with modest intakes (2–4 cups of coffee) of caffeine. In another study, elevated blood glucose levels were reported after consumption of several cups of strong coffee in a short time. However, there is not enough scientific evidence available concerning the effect of caffeine on blood glucose to recommend limiting caffeine intake for people with diabetes. Monitor your individual blood glucose response to caffeine and decide if you need to alter your consumption.

As a mild stimulant to the central nervous system, some people drink coffee just to keep alert and prevent fatigue. Excess caffeine intake may cause increased heart rate, jitters, anxiety, and insomnia. These physical effects don't last long, since caffeine doesn't accumulate in the body and is excreted within three to four hours. Drinking beverages with caffeine can be habit-forming, but not addictive. Caffeine can produce a diuretic effect, increasing water loss through urination. The more caffeine, the greater its potential for increasing water loss. This may be of concern for people at risk for dehydration.

As part of a healthy eating plan, most people can enjoy caffeine-containing beverages and food in moderation. You may consider curbing your intake if any of the following conditions apply to you.

- You experience adverse effects on your blood glucose levels.
- You have trouble sleeping and quickly get the coffee jitters.
- You're pregnant or nursing. Sensitivity to caffeine may increase during pregnancy, and caffeine can pass to the baby through the placenta and through breast milk.
- You have high blood pressure, gastritis, or ulcers. Caffeine stimulates the flow of stomach acids and can irritate the stomach.
- Caffeine-containing foods and beverages take the place of more healthy foods or beverages.

If you choose to decrease your intake of caffeine, cut back gradually to avoid problems such as headaches or drowsiness. Try a mixture of half regular and half decaffeinated coffee or drink other beverages such as water or caffeine-free herbal tea or soda.

Calories

Calories are defined as the amount of energy value in a food, as well as the amount of energy the body uses. Calories come from the three major nutrients—protein, fat, and carbohydrate—as well as alcohol. Protein and carbohydrate have 4 calories per gram, fat supplies 9 calories per gram, and alcohol has 7 calories per gram. One pound of body fat equals about 3500 calories.

The calories in our food provide the energy our body needs. The challenge for people with diabetes is to find the ideal calorie balance to maintain a reasonable weight for adults, provide for normal growth and development in children and adolescents, meet the needs of pregnancy and lactation, and recover from serious illness. The following is one method of estimating calorie needs for adults.

- **Baseline Calories:** Equals 10–12 calories per pound of desirable body weight.
- **Plus Activity Calories:** If sedentary, add 30% more calories. If moderately active, add 50% more calories. If strenuously active, add 100% more calories.

- **Adjustments:** Add 300 calories per day during pregnancy. Add 500 calories per day during lactation. Add 500 calories per day to gain one pound per week. Subtract 500 calories per day to lose one pound per week.

Your registered dietitian can help you determine your specific calorie needs based on factors such as your current calorie intake, your level of blood glucose control, and your activity level.

Carbohydrate

Carbohydrate is the primary nutrient in food that causes blood glucose to rise. Almost 90% of the carbohydrate we eat appears in the blood as glucose within two hours after we eat it. Carbohydrate is our body's major source of energy. Determining the amount of carbohydrate you can eat while keeping your blood glucose levels on target is one of the most important concepts in diabetes nutrition. Carbohydrate is found in breads, crackers, cereal, pasta, rice and other grains, dried beans, vegetables, milk and yogurt, fruit and fruit juice, table sugar, honey, syrup, and molasses, as well as foods sweetened with these items.

Certain foods such as meat, fish, eggs, oils, cheese, bacon, butter, and margarine contain little or no carbohydrate and don't raise blood glucose as much as carbohydrate-containing foods. Some foods such as cake, ice cream, candy, snack foods, pizza, casseroles, and soups contain a combination of protein, fat, and carbohydrate. Combination foods take longer to digest and may make your blood glucose rise later than you expect.

Sugars, starches, and fiber are the major types of carbohydrate. All carbohydrates are made of carbon, hydrogen, and oxygen arranged in single units. Sugars are made of one or two units (monosaccharides or disaccharides), while starches and fiber have many more (polysaccharides). In the past, you may have heard carbohydrates referred to as either "simple" (such as table sugar) or "complex" (such as potatoes) based on the number of units of carbon, hydrogen, and oxygen they contain. The term "sugars" is now used to describe simple carbohydrates and "starch" is used to describe complex carbohydrates.

Contrary to popular belief, whether a carbohydrate is made of sugars or starch has no effect on how fast the glucose produced as a result of eating it gets into the bloodstream. In the past, people with diabetes were advised to avoid sugary foods and replace them with starches. However, scientific research has found that blood glucose levels respond in the same way whether the carbohydrate comes from sugars or starches. In other words, it is more important to concentrate on the total amount of carbohydrate you eat, rather than the source of carbohydrate. Several factors influence your blood glucose response to carbohydrate, including:

- the amount of carbohydrate you eat.
- the way in which the food was cooked and processed.
- how quickly the food is digested.
- other nutrients in the food, such as fat.
- your blood glucose level at the beginning of the meal.

The amount of carbohydrate in food is measured in grams. Food labels and reference books can provide helpful information about the total carbohydrate content of foods, which is especially useful if you are using the carbohydrate counting meal planning approach (see page 34 for more information). A registered dietitian can work with you to determine the ideal amount and timing of carbohydrate in your meal plan for improved blood glucose control.

Useful References

- **Books**

  American Diabetes Association Complete Guide to Carb Counting by Hope Warshaw and Karmeen Kulkarni. Published by the American Diabetes Association, 2001.

  The Diabetes Carbohydrate and Fat Gram Guide by Lea Ann Holzmeister. Published by The American Diabetes Association, 2000.

  The Carbohydrate Counting Cookbook by Tami Ross and Patti Geil. Published by John Wiley & Sons, 1998.

Carbohydrate Counting

Foods that contain carbohydrate, such as grains, vegetables, fruit, milk, and sweets, have the most immediate impact on your blood glucose level. Eating small amounts of carbohydrate raises blood glucose somewhat; eating larger amounts of carbohydrate will raise blood glucose more. Carbohydrate counting is a meal-planning approach that determines the amount of carbohydrate you should eat at each meal and snack to keep your blood glucose level within the target range that you and your diabetes team determine. Because carbohydrate counting is very structured, plan to spend time with a registered dietitian who can assess your diabetes goals and educate you on the specifics you'll need to be successful.

All carbohydrates theoretically affect blood glucose in the same way, so the total amount of carbohydrate you eat, rather than the source of the carbohydrate, should be your first consideration when you begin to learn this approach to meal planning. Your RD will help you set a target carbohydrate goal for each meal and snack. Frequent monitoring of blood glucose will help you stay "on target" and make adjustments as needed. Food labels and reference books can help you determine the amount of carbohydrate in foods. Proper portion sizes are critical, so you'll also need some tools of the trade to get started: measuring cups and spoons, plus a food scale.

Basic carbohydrate counting stresses sources of carbohydrate, measuring the amount of carbohydrate in foods, and setting goals to eat a consistent amount of carbohydrate at each meal and snack. As you become more skilled, you will begin to find patterns in your blood glucose levels that are related to the foods you eat, the diabetes medications you use, and your physical activity. If you take multiple daily injections of insulin or use an insulin pump, you will learn about your carbohydrate-to-insulin ratio (see page 39), which will enable you to make adjustments in your insulin dosage based on the amount of carbohydrate you choose to eat. Advanced carbohydrate counting takes into consideration the fiber and protein content of a meal, fat-free foods, and special situations such as eating out.

With the help of a registered dietitian, carbohydrate counting can work for you whether you have type 1, type 2, or gestational diabetes. Although the amount of work involved may seem overwhelming at first, managing your carbohydrate intake soon becomes second nature. And good diabetes control is worth it!

Useful References

Web Sites

www.diabetes.org
www.eatright.org

Books

American Diabetes Association Complete Guide to Carb Counting by Hope Warshaw and Karmeen Kulkarni. Published by the American Diabetes Association, 2001.

The Diabetes Carbohydrate and Fat Gram Guide by Lea Ann Holzmeister. Published by the American Diabetes Association, 2000.

The Carbohydrate Counting Cookbook by Tami Ross and Patti Geil. Published by John Wiley & Sons, 1998.

Carbohydrate Loading

Carbohydrate loading is a technique used by athletes doing events of long duration to increase their storage of glycogen, a storage form of energy found in the liver and muscle tissue. Increasing storage of energy prior to the event optimizes training and performance capabilities during the event. A carbohydrate-loading regimen must be used with caution in people with diabetes, especially those taking insulin. This approach is not effective for athletes participating in activities of short duration (less than 90 minutes).

Athletes typically begin carbohydrate loading and tapering of the duration of exercise six days before an important endurance competition. Athletes double carbohydrate intake during the last three days of the loading period. If you have diabetes, you need to carefully adjust your insulin regimen and do frequent blood glucose monitoring to maintain glucose control while achieving your diabetes care goals.

During the hours before training and/or competition, endurance athletes may consume a preexercise carbohydrate meal to boost performance and endurance. For the athlete with diabetes, this preexercise carbohydrate meal may result in elevated blood insulin levels at the start of exercise. This may result in an initial lowering of the blood glucose during the first 15–20 minutes of exercise. Additional carbohydrate may be needed about 20 minutes before an event to decrease the risk of low blood glucose. Low-fat carbohydrate foods such as crackers, muffins, yogurt, or soups are good choices. Be careful not to overeat.

Ask your health care professionals for help when implementing carbohydrate loading. They can help you outline a safe and effective exercise training and competition schedule.

Useful References

Web Sites

www.diabetes-exercise.org
www.acsm.org

Books

Safe and Healthy Exercise (booklet). Published by the International Diabetes Center, 1999.

The Fitness Book for People with Diabetes. Published by the American Diabetes Association, 1994.

Carbohydrate-to-Insulin Ratio

Knowing your carbohydrate-to-insulin ratio is helpful if you manage your diabetes with multiple daily injections or an insulin pump. It enables you to determine the relationship between the insulin you take and the food you eat. The carbohydrate-to-insulin ratio is decided in consultation with a registered dietitian by determining how much fast-acting insulin you need to cover the amount of carbohydrate in a meal or snack while keeping your blood glucose within the target range. Ultimately, it can help you add more flexibility to your diet by allowing you to calculate the amount of insulin to take in circumstances when you eat more or less carbohydrate than usual.

Keeping accurate records of food, carbohydrate intake, medication, blood glucose levels, and activity is the first step in determining your carbohydrate-to-insulin ratio. The registered dietitian will review your records to find a pattern of carbohydrate intake and insulin that keeps your blood glucose in the target range. For example, if you ate 60 grams of carbohydrate at lunch, took 4 units of fast-acting insulin, and your blood glucose level stayed within the target range after the meal, the registered dietitian would divide 60 by 4, for a carbohydrate-to-insulin ratio of 15 to 1 for lunch. That is, you require 1 unit of fast-acting insulin to cover each 15 grams of carbohydrate you eat at midday.

The carbohydrate-to-insulin ratio varies from person to person and may even differ according to the nutrient content of a meal or the time of day. For example, many people have a lower carbohydrate-to-insulin ratio at breakfast than throughout the rest of the day, meaning they need more insulin to cover the carbohydrate they eat first thing in the morning. Working closely with a registered dietitian will enable you to take advantage of the valuable information gained from determining your personal carbohydrate-to-insulin ratio.

Celiac Disease

Celiac disease (also called coeliac, nontropical sprue, celiac sprue, gluten intolerant enteropathy, or gluten sensitive enteropathy) is a condition in which there is a chronic reaction to certain protein chains, commonly referred to as glutens, found in some cereal grains. This reaction causes destruction of the villi in the small intestine, which results in malabsorption of nutrients. Celiac disease is associated with other autoimmune disorders, including type 1 diabetes. Up to 10% of people with type 1 diabetes have celiac disease.

The disease can begin at any age and the onset seems to require two factors: a genetic predisposition and some kind of trigger. The trigger could be something environmental, general stress, a physical event, or a sudden infection. Blood tests and an intestinal biopsy are used to diagnose the disease. Symptoms can range from the classic features, such as diarrhea, abdominal bloating, and weakness, to bone pain, weight loss, and malnutrition. Nutrient deficiencies and lactose intolerance can develop if untreated. People with type 1 diabetes and celiac disease may have poorly controlled blood glucose and episodes of hyper- and hypoglycemia.

The only treatment for celiac disease is a gluten/prolamin-free diet. This means avoiding all products containing wheat, rye, barley, oats, and a few other lesser-known grains. Grains and starches that are safe for consumption include rice, corn, potato, arrowroot, soybean, tapioca, chickpea, nut flours, and flaxseed. The diet excludes whole grain breads and cereals that are high in fiber and fortified with many vitamins and minerals, therefore a vitamin and mineral supplement may be necessary.

The gluten/prolamin-free diet can be very challenging to follow, especially for people with diabetes. There are many hidden sources of gluten/prolamin in foods and supplements. The expertise of a registered dietitian will be needed to learn how to eliminate gluten/prolamin from the diet. The carbohydrate content of the gluten/prolamin-free grains and starches varies considerably from those containing gluten/prolamin.

Useful References

Web Sites

www.csaceliacs.org
www.celiac.com

Books

Against the Grain by Jax Peters Lowell. Published by Henry, Holt & Co., Inc., 1996.

The Gluten-Free Gourmet by Bette Hagman. Published by Henry, Holt & Co., Inc., 2000.

Certified Diabetes Educator (CDE)

A certified diabetes educator (CDE) is an invaluable resource for you as you learn the skills of diabetes self-management. A CDE may have a background as a registered nurse, registered dietitian, pharmacist, physician, physician assistant, podiatrist, exercise physiologist, physical therapist, occupational therapist, social worker, or psychologist. In addition to meeting education requirements, an individual who wishes to become a CDE must have a minimum of two calendar years experience in diabetes patient and self-management education, as well as successfully pass a certification examination on all areas of diabetes management. The National Certification Board for Diabetes Educators (NCBDE) requires that all CDEs renew their certification every five years by maintaining valid credentials in addition to passing the CDE examination.

The certification process helps to ensure that CDEs possesses distinct and specialized knowledge of diabetes, which promotes high-quality care for patients with diabetes. A CDE can help you create an individual self-management plan focusing on nutrition, monitoring, physical activity, medication, and adjusting emotionally to diabetes. You can find a certified diabetes educator through the web site of the American Association of Diabetes Educators at www.aadenet.org. To learn more about the process of becoming a CDE, access the web site of the National Certification Board for Diabetes Educators at www.ncbde.org.

Children (Ages 6–11)

School-age youngsters are establishing eating and diabetes care habits that last a lifetime. They push for independence, associate more with their peers, and make more of their own choices. Nutrition requirements for children with diabetes aged 6–11 are no different than children without diabetes. But the primary goal of the meal plan is to achieve blood glucose goals.

A major focus during these years is helping children learn to control their blood glucose levels by choosing from a wide variety of foods, staying active, and monitoring the effects with blood glucose testing. Depending on their age, many kids know the basics of healthy eating. The challenge for patents, teachers, and other adults is to help them make the link between what they know and their food choices.

As children develop their diabetes care habits, keep in mind that they will grow an average of two inches per year and gain about five pounds. Children's appetites and food preferences may change quickly. This may challenge your desire for them to follow a consistent meal plan. Carbohydrate counting with a flexible insulin schedule helps achieve blood glucose goals as appetite and physical activity levels change.

With varied appetite and physical activity levels, two to three snacks per day are often common. The number and timing of snacks will also be determined by the insulin schedule. School-age children begin to consume more meals and snacks away from home during school lunches, birthday parties, or sleepovers. This offers the opportunity for parents to help children learn guidelines for insulin and food adjustments to prevent hypoglycemia. Review school lunch menus with your child and decide how the menu can be modified if necessary. Work with school personnel to ensure that diabetes care gets the appropriate type and amount of attention needed.

Participation in organized sports, school activities, and physical education classes is common. Review meal plan changes regularly with your child and your health care professionals to incorporate appetite, exercise, and activity schedules.

Useful References

- **Web Sites**
  www.childrenwithdiabetes.com
  www.jdfcure.org

- **Books**
  Getting a Grip on Diabetes: Quick Tips & Techniques for Kids and Teens by Spike and Bo Nasmyth Loy. Published by the American Diabetes Association, 2001.

  Guide to Raising a Child with Diabetes, 2nd Edition, by Linda Siminerio and Jean Betschart. Published by the American Diabetes Association, 2000.

  Sweet Kids: How to Balance Diabetes Control & Good Nutrition with Family Peace by Betty Brackenridge and Richard Rubin. Published by the American Diabetes Association, 1996.

Cholesterol (Dietary)

Cholesterol is a waxy, fat-like substance found in foods of animal origin and in every body cell. Blood, or serum cholesterol, circulates in the bloodstream. Cholesterol is produced in your liver and also comes from food. It can never be found in foods from plant sources. That means that vegetables, fruit, beans and peas, grains, and seeds are all cholesterol free.

Limiting cholesterol intake is important because a diet high in dietary cholesterol is one factor that can elevate blood cholesterol levels for some people. However, dietary cholesterol doesn't automatically become blood cholesterol. Your total fat, especially saturated fat, has a more significant effect on blood cholesterol levels than dietary cholesterol does. The cholesterol guideline for people with diabetes is the same as for people without diabetes. Your diet should contain less than 300 milligrams of cholesterol per day. Some individuals may benefit from lowering dietary cholesterol to less than 200 mg per day.

Animal sources of foods such as meat, poultry, seafood, dairy products, butter, lard, egg yolks, and organ meats contain varying amounts of cholesterol. Some of these foods may be somewhat high in cholesterol, such as organ meats and shellfish, but be relatively low in fat and saturated fat. Keep in mind that foods of plant origin can also have cholesterol-containing ingredients such as egg yolk, milk, or butter added. It's best to check food labels for their specific cholesterol content. Foods may be labeled "no cholesterol" or "cholesterol free," which means that the product cannot contain more than 2 milligrams of cholesterol per serving. A "low cholesterol" food contains 20 milligrams or less of cholesterol. Check the Nutrition Facts panel on food labels for the cholesterol content of foods.

To decrease your intake of cholesterol, choose fat-free or low-fat dairy products, limit your total intake of meat to less than six ounces per day, and use liquid oil or soft tub margarine instead of butter or lard. Unlike dairy products, lean meat doesn't always have a low cholesterol content, because cholesterol is present in flesh as well as in fat and skin. The amount of cholesterol in a very high-fat meat, such as salami, is actually less than the amount of cholesterol in an equal amount of skinless chicken. Not that salami is a better choice—just that by limiting your total meat intake each day, you can limit your cholesterol intake as well.

Complications

The DCCT and the UKPDS studies gave us evidence that an elevated glucose level in the blood for a long time can cause diabetes complications. (See pages 64 and 240 for more information.) High blood glucose can damage many parts of the body, such as the heart, blood vessels, and kidneys. It is unclear who will get diabetes complications and when they will get them. Some people have diabetes for many years before complications arise, and some people diagnosed with diabetes as adults may already have diabetes complications. The good news is that we know how to prevent diabetes complications or slow them down.

Talk with your health care professionals about how you can be active to prevent diabetes complications.

- Keep your blood glucose and glycohemoglobin levels as close to your goal as you can. Take your diabetes medicines and check your blood glucose levels regularly.
- High blood pressure will damage your eyes, kidneys, heart, and blood vessels. You can lower your blood pressure by losing weight, exercising, and limiting the

amount of alcohol you drink. For some people, a low-sodium diet may help lower blood pressure. Your doctor may also prescribe a blood pressure medicine.

- Quit smoking. Smoking slows down the blood flow and can make heart and blood vessel problems worse. Smoking can slow blood flow to your feet and legs and make sores and infections harder to heal. If you smoke, ask your health care providers about methods that can help you quit.

- Follow a healthy eating plan that is low in cholesterol and saturated fat with lots of whole grains, fruits, and vegetables. Your meal plan can help you control your weight, keep your blood glucose levels under control, and reduce your risk for cardiovascular and kidney disease.

- Exercise regularly to improve blood glucose control and delay or prevent heart problems. Exercise can help you lose weight and improve insulin resistance.

- Check your feet every day for cuts, blisters, sores, swelling, redness, or sore toenails. Brush and floss your teeth and gums every day.

Take steps to prevent diabetes complications by following your diabetes care schedule. If you develop diabetes complications, seek up-to-date information on treatments and prevention. Understand what causes the complications and how you can prevent them from getting worse. (See pages 133 and 161 for more information on heart disease and kidney disease.)

- Diabetes eye disease is sometimes called **retinopathy**. High blood glucose and high blood pressure from diabetes can damage the blood vessels that supply blood to the retina in your eyes. Retinas have tiny blood vessels that are easy to damage. As diabetes retina problems get worse, new blood vessels in the retina grow. These new blood vessels are weak and can break easily, causing vision problems.

- Diabetes nerve disease is sometimes called **neuropathy**. High blood glucose levels over a long period of time can damage your nervous system by causing nerve damage and poor blood flow. Nerve damage can cause pain in your hands, feet, thighs, and face. It can cause trouble with digestion or bladder or bowel control. It may even cause types of sexual dysfunction.

Useful References

- **Web Site**
  www.niddk.nih.gov

- **Book**
  The Uncomplicated Guide to Diabetes Complications by Marvin E. Levin and Michael A. Pfeifer. Published by the American Diabetes Association, 1998.

Constipation

Constipation is the inability to move food smoothly through the gastrointestinal tract, resulting in a decrease in frequency of bowel movements, the presence of hard stool, or the need for straining. It is by far the most common gastrointestinal complication of diabetes. Constipation may be related to the diabetic complication neuropathy, or nerve damage to the intestine. Or, it could simply be due to poor eating habits, lack of physical activity, and inadequate fluid intake.

If you find yourself experiencing frequent bouts of constipation, see your physician to investigate the underlying cause—you may need medication. The following tips may also help activate a sluggish bowel.

- Drink at least 8 cups of liquid a day, such as water or sugar-free or calorie-free drinks.
- Be sure to eat plenty of fiber from sources such as whole grains, fruits, and vegetables. However, check with your physician before embarking on a very high-fiber diet. Some types of fiber can slow the movement of stools through the gastrointestinal tract, causing fecal im-

paction. If you have gastroparesis, also known as "stomach paralysis," a high-fiber intake can even be harmful.

- Stay physically active, which will help intestinal movement.
- Avoid strong laxatives; your body may become dependent on them. Stool softeners or psyllium supplements are available over the counter and may be effective when combined with the other tips mentioned above.

Convenience Foods

Convenience foods are foods that require little or no preparation before eating. With the busy pace of life today, these foods have become commonplace in many households. Though convenience foods have not always been in line with the goals for healthy eating, markets are adding new meal solutions and shortcuts that can meet your nutrition and health needs. With mindful planning, convenience foods can be a healthy answer to those last-minute meal crunches.

An increase in the variety and types of convenience foods offers even more opportunities to save you time in meal planning and preparation. Labor- and step-saving ingredients such as pizza crust or bread dough can save you time and money, since you don't need to keep supplies of ingredients on hand that you rarely use. Precut, cleaned ready-to-cook vegetables, precut cleaned and bagged salads, and frozen foods are the most frequent convenience items purchased by shoppers. Supermarket take-out foods found in salad bars or delis can also be healthy timesaving options. Refrigerated or frozen fully cooked meat entrees such as pot roasts and chicken fillets can be assembled with convenience side items to make a meal in a flash.

Select convenience foods that meet your nutrition goals by using these healthy food selection guidelines.

- Does the food fit with my health goals?
- Does the food satisfy one or more of my dietary goals?
- Will this food help me follow my meal plan or will it sabotage it?
- How often do I eat this food?
- Compared with similar products on the shelf, how does it stack up nutritionally?
- Does it have more fat, salt, and sugar than other nutrients?

Useful Reference

- **Book**
  Complete Guide to Convenience Food Counts by Lea Ann Holzmeister. Published by the American Diabetes Association, 2001.

Conventional Therapy

Conventional therapy is a system of diabetes management practiced by many people with diabetes. This approach to therapy usually applies to people with type 1 diabetes and consists of one or two insulin injections each day, daily self-monitoring of blood glucose, and a standard program of nutrition and exercise. The main objective of treatment is to avoid very high and very low blood glucose levels.

In two well-known studies, the DCCT and the UKPDS, a comparison of conventional therapy and intensive therapy showed that the risk for diabetes complications was decreased with lowering blood glucose using intensive therapy. (See pages 64 and 240 for more information.) The American Diabetes Association recommends treatment of diabetes aimed at lowering blood glucose to or near normal level in all people with diabetes.

With conventional insulin therapy of twice-daily injections of short- and intermediate-acting insulin before breakfast and the evening meal, the timing of food intake should be synchronized with the administration of insulin. Consistency in the timing and amount of food intake is important.

Treatment approaches for diabetes should take into account your ability to understand and carry out the treatment regimen as well as the resources available to you. The type and amount of diabetes medicines you take, your meal plan, and your monitoring schedule will depend on factors such as type of diabetes, stage of the disease (type 2), and blood glucose goals. Discuss your diabetes management goals with your health care providers. They will help you determine the best approach to your successful diabetes management.

Useful References

- **Web Site**
  www.diabetes.org

- **Books**
  American Diabetes Association Complete Guide to Diabetes, 2nd Edition. Published by the American Diabetes Association, 1999.

  Diabetes A to Z, 4th Edition. Published by the American Diabetes Association, 2000.

Cow's Milk

Different kinds of foods have been implicated in the development of type 1 diabetes. Researchers have studied the link between short periods, or absence, of breastfeeding and increased incidence of type 1 diabetes. Use of cow's milk-based infant formulas has been suspect. Children with type 1 diabetes have shown higher amounts of antibodies that recognize a specific protein in cow's milk. The immune response to the milk proteins might be related to the destruction of insulin-producing beta cells in the pancreas in certain genetically susceptible children. Other studies have shown that there is no association between cow's milk and beta-cell autoimmunity.

Research has shown that human milk and breastfeeding of infants provide advantages with regard to general health, growth, and development, while significantly decreasing risk for a large number of acute and chronic diseases. Breast milk is the best source of nutrition during the first year of life for infants with or without diabetes. The baby benefits even when breastfed for only a short time.

Cow's milk is only one kind of food that may play a role in the development of type 1 diabetes. Commercial infant formula is a healthy alternative or supplement to breastfeeding. The cow's milk used to make infant formula has been modified to meet an infant's special needs. Deciding to breastfeed is a personal decision made with your partner and your pediatrician, who can assimilate the current research and discuss options with you in a fully informed manner. Discuss questions or concerns with your diabetes professionals and your pediatrician.

DASH Diet

The DASH diet is a very successful nutrition approach to improving high blood pressure. Scientific studies show that individuals with high blood pressure who followed the DASH diet lowered their systolic pressure on average about 11 mm/Hg and diastolic pressure about 6 mm/Hg, without medication, within two weeks of starting the eating plan. Recent research also shows that the DASH diet significantly reduces the levels of total cholesterol and of low-density lipoproteins (LDLs) or "bad" cholesterol.

DASH stands for Dietary Approaches to Stop Hypertension and is the name for an eating plan that was developed as part of a study funded by the National Institutes of Health. The DASH diet is:

- high in fruits and vegetables
- high in low-fat dairy products
- high in fiber
- one that contains about 3000 mg of sodium per day (although more dramatic blood pressure lowering occurs if sodium is reduced to 1500 mg per day)
- low in fat and saturated fat

A 2000-calorie DASH eating plan recommends daily servings as follows:

- 7–8 servings of grains and grain products
- 4–5 servings of vegetables
- 4–5 servings of fruits
- 2–3 servings of low-fat dairy products
- 2 or fewer servings of meats, poultry, and fish
- 2–3 servings of fats and oils

In addition, weekly intake of 4–5 servings of nuts, seeds, and dry beans and no more than 5 servings of sweets is recommended.

The DASH eating plan has not been specifically tested in people with diabetes. If you have high blood pressure, talk with your physician and registered dietitian to determine if the DASH diet principles can be applied to your current meal plan.

Useful Reference

- **Web Site**
  www.dash.bwh.harvard.edu

Dehydration/Fluid Requirements

Every day you lose an amount of water equal to about 4% of your total weight. If you do not take in enough water to replace what you lose naturally by breathing, perspiring, and urinating, symptoms of dehydration can set in. Inadequate fluid intake during extreme temperatures or strenuous work or exercise can lead to depleted body water.

Poorly controlled diabetes, medications, and illness can also cause dehydration. Elevated blood glucose causes the kidneys to increase urine production, which can lead to dehydration. Certain medications, such as diuretics and antibiotics, interact with body fluids and affect water requirements. Repeated vomiting, diarrhea, or high fevers can drain your body of water and electrolytes. In the older person, a diminished level of consciousness and thirst perception, fluid restrictions, and aging kidneys can cause dehydration.

The effects of dehydration, or loss of body water, are progressive. The first signal of dehydration is thirst. If you ignore thirst it will just get more intense. Eventually your appetite fades and you experience fatigue, weakness, headaches, nausea, and flushing. At this point you are in danger of spiraling quickly into severe symptoms of dehydration.

To keep your body functioning normally and to avoid dehydration, your body needs an ongoing water supply. Most people need 8 to 12 cups of water daily from drinking water, other beverages, and water in solid foods. For strenuous work or exercise, drink one to three more cups per hour. When you are sick, taking medication, or have an elevated blood glucose level, follow the advice of your health care provider and drink plenty of water and other fluids to prevent dehydration.

Diabetes Control and Complications Trial (DCCT)

The Diabetes Control and Complications Trial (DCCT) was a landmark study conducted over seven years in patients with type 1 diabetes that proved that the complications of diabetes are related to high blood glucose levels. Two groups of patients were followed long term. One group was treated conventionally, with the standard forms of treatment and blood glucose goals, and one was treated intensively, where the goal for each patient was to achieve normal blood glucose levels.

Although not all patients in the intensive treatment group were able to achieve normal blood glucose, overall there were improvements in hemoglobin A_{1c} and blood glucose values. The intensive treatment group also showed a 60% reduction in the risk of diabetes complications including eye disease, kidney disease, and nerve complications.

To achieve these levels of blood glucose control, intensively treated patients required multiple (three or more) insulin injections daily or treatment with an insulin pump. Intensively treated patients did have an increased risk of hypoglycemia and experienced significant weight gain.

Although the DCCT was not designed to be a "diet study," the patients in the conventional treatment group saw a registered dietitian every six months; those in the intensive treatment group saw the RD at least twice as often, once every three months. Each research center in the study decided on its own method of meal planning, from *Exchange Lists for Meal Planning* to *Dietary Guidelines for Americans* to carbohydrate counting. The positive results proved that no single meal plan works for everyone, just as no single medication is effective for everyone with diabetes. An individualized assessment by a registered dietitian is the best way to select from the variety of meal planning options to find the one that will work for you.

The United Kingdom Prospective Diabetes Study (UKPDS) demonstrated that improved blood glucose control in patients with type 2 diabetes reduces the risk of developing eye and kidney complications and possibly reduces nerve complications. (See page 240 for more information.)

Diabetes Food Pyramid

The Diabetes Food Pyramid was developed by the American Diabetes Association and The American Dietetic Association as a slight modification of the Food Guide Pyramid developed by the United States Department of Agriculture. The pyramid concept is a tool to put the *Dietary Guidelines for Americans* into action. There are six food groups with foods you should eat more of towards the bottom of the pyramid. The food pyramid is helpful as an introduc-

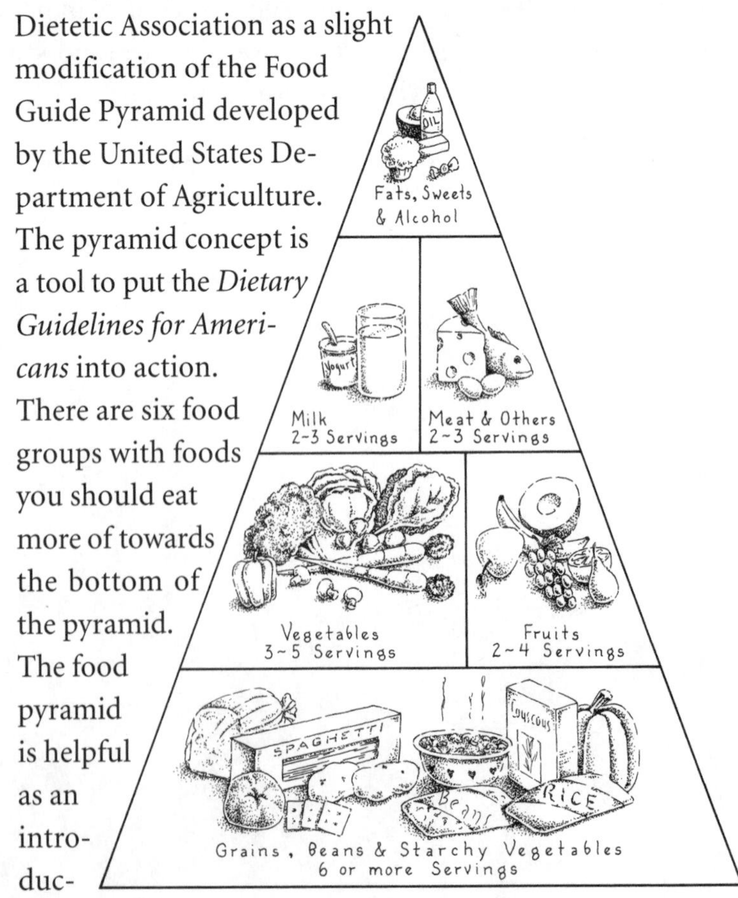

tion to basic nutrition. It may be the only information you need to improve your eating habits and diabetes control. However, you may want to work with your registered dietitian to modify the pyramid into a more structured approach to meal planning.

The diabetes food pyramid calls for eating a variety of foods to get the nutrients you need, with the right amount of calories to maintain or improve your weight.

- **Grains, Beans, and Starchy Vegetables Group:** Sample serving sizes from this group include 1 slice of bread, 1/3 cup cooked beans, or 1/2 cup of cooked cereal or pasta. Foods from this group provide an important source of energy, especially if you are limiting your fat. They also provide vitamins, minerals, and fiber.

- **Vegetable Group:** Sample serving sizes from this group are 1 cup of raw vegetables, 1/2 cup of cooked vegetables, or 1/2 cup of vegetable juice. Vegetables provide vitamins such as vitamins A, C, and folate and minerals such as iron and magnesium. They are low in fat and also provide fiber.

- **Fruit Group:** A fruit serving is considered to be a small apple or banana, 1/2 cup of cooked or canned fruit, or 1/2 cup of fruit juice. Fruits and juices provide important amounts of vitamins A, C, and potassium, as well as being low in fat and sodium.

- **Meat and Others Group:** Two to 3 ounces of cooked lean meat, poultry, or fish count as a serving. Other food serving sizes in the group include 1 egg or 1 tablespoon of peanut butter. The foods from this group provide protein, B vitamins, iron, and zinc.

- **Milk Group:** A serving from this group may be 1 cup of milk or 3/4 cup of plain nonfat yogurt. Milk products are the best source of calcium, in addition to providing protein, vitamins, and other minerals.

- **Fats, Sweets, and Alcohol:** The small tip of the pyramid shows foods such as salad dressings and oils, cream, butter, margarine, sugars, soft drinks, candies, sweet desserts, and alcohol. While these foods provide calories, they are otherwise nutritionally empty. Use with caution!

A 2200-calorie diet for a person with diabetes would include the following food servings per day.

- **Grains, Beans, and Starchy Vegetables Group:** 6 or more servings
- **Vegetable Group:** 3–5 servings
- **Fruit Group:** 2–4 servings
- **Meat and Others Group:**
  2–3 servings
- **Milk Group:** 2–3 servings
- **Fats, Sweets, and Alcohol:** use sparingly

No matter which meal planning approach you use, stick with the goal of reaching your target blood glucose and blood lipid levels!

Useful References

- **Web Site**
  www.diabetes.org
- **Book**
  Diabetes Meal Planning Made Easy: How to Put the Food Pyramid to Work for You, 2nd Edition, by Hope Warshaw. Published by the American Diabetes Association, 2000.

Dietary Guidelines for Americans

The 5th Edition of the *Dietary Guidelines for Americans* was released in May 2000 as a joint publication of the Departments of Health and Human Services and Agriculture. While these guidelines aren't written specifically for people with diabetes, they are the most up-to-date advice from nutrition scientists and should be the basis of any diabetes meal planning approach you use. The guidelines are listed below.

- **Aim for Fitness**
  - Aim for a healthy weight.
  - Be physically active each day.
- **Build a Healthy Base**
  - Let the food pyramid guide your food choices.
  - Choose a variety of grains daily, especially whole grains.
  - Choose a variety of fruits and vegetables daily.
  - Keep food safe to eat.
- **Choose Sensibly**
  - Choose a diet that is low in saturated fat and cholesterol and moderate in total fat.

- Choose beverages and foods to moderate your intake of sugars.
- Choose and prepare foods with less salt.
- If you drink alcoholic beverages, do so in moderation.

Useful Reference

- **Web Site**
  www.health.gov/dietaryguidelines/

Dietary Reference Intakes (DRIs)

Dietary Reference Intakes (DRIs) are reference values that are quantitative estimates of recommended nutrient intakes for vitamins, minerals, and other nutrients like fiber, protein, and fat. In the past, Recommended Daily Allowances (RDAs) were widely recognized as the benchmark of nutritional adequacy. DRIs were developed in response to the dramatic increase in scientific knowledge about the role of nutrients in prevention of disease and nutritional deficiencies.

DRI is a generic term that refers to at least four types of reference nutrient values: Recommended Dietary Allowance, Adequate Intake, Tolerable Upper Intake Level, and Estimated Average Requirement.

- **Recommended Dietary Allowance (RDA)** is the average daily dietary intake level that is sufficient to meet the nutrient requirement of nearly all (97–98%) healthy individuals in a particular life stage and gender group.
- **Adequate Intake (AI)** is a recommended intake value based on observed or experimentally determined approximations or estimates of nutrient intake by a

group (or groups) of healthy people that are assumed to be adequate. The AI is used when an RDA cannot be determined.

- **Tolerable Upper Intake Level (UL)** is the highest level of daily nutrient intake that is likely to pose no risk of adverse health effects for almost all individuals in the general population. As intake increases above the UL, the risk of adverse effects may increase.
- **Estimated Average Requirement (EAR)** is a daily nutrient intake value that is estimated to meet the requirement of half of the healthy individuals in a life stage or gender group.

Since 1993, DRIs have been a work in progress. The Food and Nutrition Board of the National Academy of Sciences is constantly researching nutrients and making new recommendations as the information becomes available. Thus far, the DRI Panels have reported new recommendations for calcium, phosphorus, magnesium, fluoride, thiamin, riboflavin, niacin, vitamin B6, folate, vitamin B12, pantothenic acid, biotin, choline, vitamin C, vitamin E, beta-carotene, vitamin A, vitamin K, and a number of trace minerals including selenium and vanadium.

While DRIs are not published on nutrition facts food panels or on vitamin/mineral supplement bottles, there is a general relationship with the Percent Daily Values. Contact your registered dietitian for your nutrient recommendations or visit the web site below.

Useful Reference

- **Web Site**
  www.nationalacademies.org.

Diverticulosis

Diverticulosis is a common condition in middle-aged and elderly people in which tiny protruding pouches (diverticula) are present in the colon. These pouches are like an inner tube that pokes through weak places in a tire. When the pouches become infected or inflamed, the condition is called diverticulitis. It is believed that diverticular disease is caused by a low-fiber diet. This can lead to constipation, making the muscles strain to move stool that is too hard. This can cause increased pressure in the colon and weak spots that bulge out and become diverticula.

Most people with diverticulitis do not have any discomfort or symptoms. However, the inflammation might cause mild cramps, bloating, and constipation. You should visit your doctor if you have any of these symptoms. The most common symptom of diverticulitis is abdominal pain or tenderness around the left side of the lower abdomen. If an infection is present, fever, nausea, vomiting, chills, constipation, and cramping may occur. Contact your physician if these symptoms are present.

The treatment for diverticular disease is a high-fiber diet, and occasionally pain medications. Fiber keeps stools soft and lowers the pressure inside the colon so that bowel contents can move through easily. Many experts recommend 20–35 grams of fiber each day. (See page 101 for more information on fiber.) Your physician may also recommend drinking a fiber product such as Citrucel or Metamucil once a day. Many doctors have suggested avoiding foods with small seeds such as tomatoes or strawberries because they believed that particles could lodge in the diverticula and cause inflammation. However, this remains controversial and no evidence supports this recommendation.

The treatment for diverticulitis focuses on clearing up the infection and inflammation, resting the colon, and preventing or minimizing complications. Your doctor may ask you to follow a liquid diet to help your colon rest. He or she might recommend pain relievers and antibiotics to control the muscle spasms in your colon and treat the infection. If attacks are severe or frequent, your physician may advise surgical intervention.

For more information, contact the National Digestive Disease Information Clearinghouse at the National Institute of Diabetes, Digestive, and Kidney Disease (NIDDK) at the web site below.

Useful Reference

- **Web Site**
  www.niddk.nih.gov

Eating Disorders

The problem of eating disorders in people with diabetes has received much attention in the past few years. It is unclear whether eating disorders occur more frequently in people with diabetes than the rest of the population. But people with diabetes who are necessarily preoccupied with issues of food, diet, and weight control can be more vulnerable to developing eating disorders.

There are two general types of eating disorders: anorexia nervosa and bulimia nervosa. Though the causes of anorexia and bulimia are not fully understood, they are actually distorted eating habits, often related to emotional problems. Usually there is a negative self-image and struggles with depression and other psychological problems. Frequently, the person's whole life—schoolwork or career, family life, day-to-day patterns, emotions, growth, overall health—gets wrapped up in eating issues. Diabetes can add to this preoccupation, even obsession, with food and weight.

Anorexia typically results in low body weight, caused by an obsession with food, weight, and thinness. People suffering with anorexia deny hunger and refuse to eat in order to stay thin. They may exercise excessively and show abnormal weight loss in a short time span. By starving themselves, they consume too few calories for their basic needs and their bodies slowly waste away. Anorexia leads to menstrual irregularities, osteoporosis in women, and greater risk of early death in women and men. For the person with diabetes, anorexia can cause low blood glucose levels most of the time, and hospitalization may be required for recurrent and severe bouts of hypoglycemia. Those with anorexia may lower their insulin dose to match their lower food intake.

Bulimia is marked by binge eating and purging. Underlying emotional problems, plus an intense fear of gaining weight, leads bulimics to gorge on large amounts of food (usually several thousand calories of food at one sitting or over a few hours) then purge it out of their systems by inducing vomiting or taking laxatives. Health consequences of bulimia are serious: dehydration, organ damage, internal bleeding from the stress of vomiting, tooth decay from acids in vomit, and in some cases, death.

Diabetes offers another possible form of purging. By reducing or omitting insulin after binges, people with bulimia and diabetes can drive up their blood sugar, causing calories to be lost in the urine. Many people who try this are overweight. In an attempt to control blood glucose levels, a person with bulimia may take more insulin after a binge to cover the large amount of food. Judging the absorption rate of the food and the amount of insulin needed for the binge is difficult and often leads to erratic blood glucose levels.

When eating disorders and diabetes occur together, the consequences are very serious. In addition to the typical health risks of eating disorders, people with diabetes and eating disorders are almost always in poor metabolic control, with more episodes of ketoacidosis and hypoglycemia, and their glycated hemoglobin tends to be higher. An unhealthy blood glucose level over a long period of time creates a great risk for diabetic complications that can affect every system of the body.

If you suspect that you have an eating disorder or that a friend or family member with diabetes has, don't wait until a severe weight loss or a serious diabetes complication proves you are right. Ask your primary physician to recommend a mental health professional who can work with the other members of the health care team. Treatment for an eating disorder combines medical, psychological, and nutritional counseling. Participation in support groups as well as group counseling for family members is an important part of treatment.

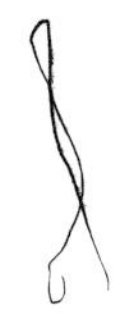

Eggs

Eggs are part of the Meat Group on the Diabetes Food Guide Pyramid and supply protein, iron, and vitamins A, D, and B12. They can be an economical and convenient source of high-quality protein. To control blood cholesterol and heart disease, you should eat less than 300 milligrams of cholesterol every day (less than 200 milligrams a day if your LDL cholesterol is greater than 100 mg/dl). As a way to control dietary cholesterol intake, health experts advise eating no more than four egg yolks a week. Egg yolks are high in cholesterol; each contains about 213 milligrams. Egg yolks are often found in processed foods and many baked goods.

Egg whites contain no cholesterol and can be used in place of whole eggs in many foods. For most cake, cookie, bread, pancake, casserole, French toast, cheesecake, pudding, and other recipes that call for whole eggs, you can use two egg whites in place of one whole egg. Since cholesterol-free liquid egg substitutes are made mainly of egg white, they also may be used to replace eggs (all or some) in dishes that call for two or more eggs such as scrambled eggs, omelets, and quiche. This maintains the color and flavor of the yolk in the recipe, but supplies less cholesterol. Egg substitutes can be found in the frozen foods aisle or refrigerated dairy section of the grocery store.

If not handled properly, eggs and egg substitutes provide the perfect medium for salmonella, a dangerous bacteria, to grow. Remember to cook eggs until they are done and keep them at 40–140 degrees for not longer than two hours. Otherwise, keep them refrigerated. Avoid foods with raw eggs such as homemade ice cream, mayonnaise, or eggnog unless they are made with a freshly opened carton of pasteurized eggs.

HOW EGGS ADD UP

Egg Product	Milligrams of Cholesterol (mg)
Omelet, 2-egg (1)	426
Cheese soufflé (1 cup)	107
Pound cake (1/12 of 9 × 9-inch cake)	107
Chocolate, lemon meringue, or pumpkin pie (1/8 of 9-inch pie)	71
Cornbread (1/9 of 9 × 9-inch pan)	53
Eggnog (about 1/2 cup)	53
Pancake, 4-inch (2)	53
Mayonnaise (2 Tbsp)	27
Yellow or chocolate two-layer cake (1/16 of 9-inch cake)	27
Muffin (1)	21

Elderly

As we age, we become more prone to developing impaired glucose tolerance and diabetes. Almost one in five adults over the age of 60 has diabetes. You may find that managing your diabetes is more difficult during this stage of life because of the additional challenges of aging: loss of support systems; other chronic conditions such as heart disease, arthritis, and hypertension; limitations in physical activity; and tighter financial resources.

Although you may face additional diabetes challenges because you are older, the basic principles of diabetes nutrition management are the same for you as for younger people. The registered dietitian on your diabetes team should do a thorough assessment of your nutrition and medical history as well as your diabetes goals and help you set personalized blood glucose targets. Monitoring your weight is also crucial, since an unexplained weight change of more than 10 pounds in less than six months can indicate problems with your nutrition status.

Your diabetes meal plan should be based on the same nutrition recommendations followed by younger people but tailored to your special needs. You may need a daily multivitamin supplement with calcium, particularly if you have a poor appetite and your calorie intake is low. If you find it difficult to cook in small amounts just for yourself, ask your dietitian for recipe and cookbook suggestions for quick and nutritious meals. Physical activity and blood glucose monitoring should remain an important part of your diabetes management plan. Paying special attention to your diabetes will help you feel well and stay healthy.

Useful References

- **Books**

Diabetic Cooking for Seniors by Kathleen Stanley. Published by the American Diabetes Association, 2001.

Quick and Easy Diabetic Recipes for One by Kathleen Stanley and Connie Crawley. Published by the American Diabetes Association, 1997.

Electrolytes

The electrolytes sodium, potassium, and chloride regulate body fluids in and out of every cell, and they transmit nerve, or electrical, impulses. They send messages from your brain to your muscles, causing them to relax or contract. For people with diabetes, the requirements for electrolytes are the same as for the general population, unless kidney disease or high blood pressure is present.

Sodium and chloride mostly work outside the cells and potassium works mainly inside the cells to help maintain fluid balance. Maintaining fluid balance is important to help your muscles, including your heart muscle, contract and relax. When you perspire during exercise, your body loses small amounts of electrolytes. In most cases you can replace sodium and other electrolytes just with foods you normally eat. Elite athletes who sweat heavily for long periods may need to replace electrolytes with sports drinks or salty foods.

For people with diabetes, maintaining electrolyte and fluid balance is important during illness to prevent dehydration and electrolyte depletion. Signs of electrolyte depletion are muscle weakness and fatigue. During illness, drinking 8 ounces of fluid every hour is recommended to prevent dehydration. Sports drinks, bouillon, consommé, and canned clear soups provide sodium and electrolytes as well as fluids.

Though there is no Recommended Dietary Allowance for potassium, the minimum amount suggested for adults is 2000 milligrams a day; some experts suggest more, about 3500 milligrams per day, to help protect against high blood pressure. Vegetables, fruits, fresh meat, poultry, and fish are among the best sources of potassium. Though a potassium deficiency is rare, when vomiting, diarrhea, and laxative use go on for too long, or there is kidney disease, the body may lose excess amounts. Weakness, appetite loss, nausea, and fatigue are symptoms of potassium deficiency.

If you are taking medication to manage high blood pressure, you may need a potassium supplement. Potassium may be restricted in your diet if you have end-stage renal disease. Potassium chloride is a salt substitute and is sometimes used when sodium is restricted. It may be harmful and is not recommended unless used under your physician's supervision.

Salt is made of sodium and chloride so salt and salty foods are the main sources of chloride. This makes a chloride deficiency unlikely. For healthy people, the Dietary Guidelines and the American Heart Association suggest a sodium intake of less than 2400 milligrams per day. Check with your health care professional about your sodium needs. (See page 216 for more information.)

Ethnic Foods

Diabetes disproportionately affects ethnic minority populations in the United States. Each ethnic group has its own culturally based (or ethnic) foods and food habits. These traditional food habits may be modified or evolve through contact with other cultures. For example, many people believe that foods that are commonly served in Chinese restaurants in the United States, such as fried chicken wings and egg rolls, are typical Chinese foods. Such dishes, however, were invented for the American palate. The indigenous Chinese diet is abundant in complex carbohydrates and includes a wide variety of meat, poultry, seafood, fruits, and vegetables.

As America becomes increasingly multi-cultural, so too does our palate. New waves of immigrants from Latin America, Asia, and the Middle East offer a new influence on foods Americans eat. Regional specialties within the United States have developed based on native foods that are available. For example, bean burritos and fish tacos have become favorites in the southwest. Restaurants and supermarkets also give us exposure to ethnic cuisines by offering new flavors and foods.

It is important to consider cultural food habits when developing your diabetes eating plan. Discuss with your dietitian how familiar foods that are culturally acceptable can be part of your meal plan. If you occasionally cook or eat ethnic foods in restaurants, learn how these foods affect your diabetes. Many traditional ethnic foods can offer health benefits, especially those that focus on grains, vegetables, legumes, and fruits.

If you are unfamiliar with menu items when ordering ethnic foods in restaurants, ask your waiter to describe the food, its ingredients, and method of preparation. Get to know the menu terms and cooking basics, especially if you need to control calories, fat, and other nutrients. Look for foods with simple preparation, such as steamed vegetables or broiled chicken. Look for menu items typically prepared with less fat or balance a higher-fat item with lower-fat choices for the rest of the meal.

The expanding multicultural palate in restaurants, supermarkets, and your own kitchen offers the opportunity to expand the variety in your eating style and stretch your food experience.

Exchange Lists for Meal Planning

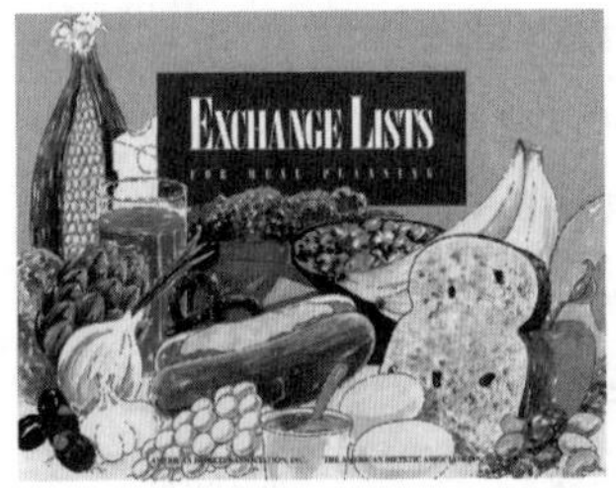

For many years, *Exchange Lists for Meal Planning* was the only meal planning resource available for people with diabetes. Over the years, it has evolved to reflect changes in nutrition knowledge for diabetes and foods available in the marketplace. However, its basic premise remains the same: foods are grouped together with other foods of similar nutrient composition, so that foods on each list can be substituted or "exchanged" with other foods on the same list. Within each food list, one exchange in the serving size described is approximately equal to another in calories, carbohydrate, protein, and fat.

The latest version of *Exchange Lists for Meal Planning* categorizes foods into the three main groups below.

- **Carbohydrate Group:** This group includes the starch, fruit, milk, "other carbohydrate," and vegetable lists. Foods from these lists can be interchanged in your meal plan, since each group contains roughly equal amounts of calories and carbohydrate.

- **Meat and Meat Substitute Group:** This group includes sources of protein and fat, divided into the very lean, lean, medium-fat, and high-fat lists.

- **Fat Group:** Familiar fats are divided into lists of monounsaturated, polyunsaturated, and saturated fats.

In addition, *Exchange Lists for Meal Planning* includes vegetarian foods, fast foods, free foods, and combination foods, and special symbols indicating foods that are high in sodium.

A registered dietitian can help you become familiar with *Exchange Lists for Meal Planning* and help you individualize it to your diabetes treatment plan. An RD can review your nutrition and health history, calculate the appropriate amount of calories and carbohydrate you need, and make an individualized meal plan for you, as well as help you establish blood glucose and eating goals.

Exchange lists are helpful in other meal planning methods such as carbohydrate choice or gram counting or fat gram counting. While following the *Exchange Lists for Meal Planning* is a structured approach, there is also a variety of other approaches available that an RD can help you choose from to improve your blood glucose control.

Useful References

- **Web Sites**
  www.diabetes.org
  www.eatright.org

Exercise (Physical Activity)

The benefits of physical activity are almost too good to be true. It can improve your physical health and emotional well-being. Exercise reduces your risk of developing coronary heart disease, which is important for anyone, but especially for people with diabetes. Exercise helps to decrease blood cholesterol and increase levels of high-density lipoprotein (HDL) cholesterol (the good cholesterol) in the blood. Physical activity can help prevent high blood pressure and reduce blood pressure in some people with hypertension. Being fit helps maintain healthy bones, muscles, and joints and reduces symptoms of anxiety and depression.

If you have diabetes, exercising can help lower blood glucose and help your body use insulin better. If you treat your diabetes with insulin, this could mean that you use less insulin. For people with type 2 diabetes, exercise combined with a healthy meal plan could mean that you can control your diabetes without the use of insulin or oral agents, or that you can get by with less medication. Exercise helps control weight, develop lean muscle, and reduce body fat, which is important for everyone, but especially for people with type 2 diabetes.

Check with your physician and other members of your health care team before you begin a new exercise program. Get your team to do a complete history and physical examination and help you develop a safe exercise plan. Talk with your registered dietitian about adjusting your eating plan, and talk with your physician about adjusting your medications to keep your blood glucose levels in control.

Make sure your exercise plan includes key ingredients to optimize the health benefits and effect on your diabetes control. A good workout session includes anything that gets your heart beating and uses the large muscles in your legs and arms. Some examples include walking, aerobics, running, swimming, water aerobics, stair climbing, bike riding, or dancing. Start your workout with 5–10 minutes of warm-up exercises and stretching. Follow this with 20–30 minutes of aerobic activity. Follow your exercise with 5–10 minutes of cool-down exercises and stretching.

To experience the benefits of exercise, plan your workouts for most days of the week. A good time to exercise is one to three hours after a meal or snack. The meal or snack will help keep your blood glucose from falling too low. Check with your health care provider about the best time for your workouts. If you take insulin or oral diabetes medications that may cause low blood glucose, you may need a snack before, during, or after you exercise. If you are trying to lose weight, talk to your health care team about using less insulin or medicine instead of eating more food. The type and amount of snacks you take will depend on your blood glucose before you exercise and how long and hard you will be exercising.

If your blood glucose is more than 240 mg/dl, and you take insulin, test your urine for ketones. (See page 159 for more information.) If you show moderate or large ketone levels, this means you do not have enough insulin. You may need another insulin injection. Do not exercise until ketone levels return to negative or trace amounts. Follow the guidelines below for maintaining your blood glucose while exercising.

- **30 minutes of low intensity exercise** (walking): If blood glucose is less than 100 mg/dl before exercise, eat a snack with 15 grams of carbohydrate.
- **30–60 minutes of moderate intensity exercise** (tennis, swimming, jogging): If blood glucose is less than 100 mg/dl before exercise, have a snack with 25–50 grams of carbohydrate. If blood glucose is 100–180 mg/dl, eat 10–15 grams of carbohydrate.
- **1–2 hours of strenuous intensity exercise** (basketball, skiing, shoveling snow): If blood glucose is less than 100 mg/dl before exercise, add a snack with about 50 grams of carbohydrate. If blood glucose is 100–180 mg/dl, add a snack with 25–50 grams of carbohydrate. If blood glucose is 180–250 mg/dl, have a snack with 10–15 grams of carbohydrate. At this intense level of exercise, always monitor blood glucose carefully.

Here are some suggested snacks that contain about 15 grams of carbohydrate each.

- 1/2 cup fruit juice (can be diluted)
- 1 small piece of fruit
- 1 cup yogurt
- 1/2 English muffin or bagel
- 1 small muffin
- 1 cup yogurt
- 2 Tbsp raisins
- 6–8 oz sports drink
- 4–5 snack crackers
- 1/4 cup dried fruit
- 1/2 snack bar

When you are exercising, don't wait to be thirsty to drink plenty of fluids. Dehydration can hinder your strength and endurance. Cool water is the best fluid to drink if you are exercising for less than 60 minutes. Avoid soft drinks with caffeine. These can contribute to dehydration. If you exercise for more than 60 minutes, diluted fruit juice or a sports drink can be useful to replace fluids and minerals and keep your blood glucose in the normal range.

Aerobic exercise makes you breathe harder and your heart beat faster. This burns calories and increases your body's rate of metabo-

	Body Weight	
Activity (30 minutes)	**120 lbs**	**170 lbs**
Aerobic dance, low impact	140	195
Aerobic dance, high impact	195	270
Bowling	85	115
Construction work, outside	150	210
Cycling, leisure	165	230
Cycling, stationary, moderate effort	195	270
Dancing	125	175
Golf (walking)	125	175
Gardening	140	195
Housework	70	95
Home repair	85	115
Hunting	140	195
Ice skating	195	270
Jogging	195	270
Mowing lawn	150	215
Racquetball	195	270
Skiing	195	270
Swimming, moderate laps	220	310
Tai Chi	110	155
Tennis	195	270
Walking, brisk (4 mph)	110	155
Water aerobics	110	155
Yoga	110	155

lism for several hours after the exercise. This can lead to delayed hypoglycemia. Check your blood glucose before and after exercise and during long, hard exercise. Muscles keep burning glucose even after you stop exercising. It may take the body up to 24 hours to replace glucose stores used during exercise. After strenuous exercise, you may need to monitor your blood glucose every 1–2 hours.

For people trying to lose weight, exercise offers a double bonus, the ability to burn calories at the time of exercise and hours later. Refer to the table on the previous page for calories burned in various physical activities.

Useful References

- **Web Site**

  www.diabetes-exercise.org

- **Books**

  Diabetes Day-by-Day: Starting to Exercise and 20 Steps to Safe Exercise. Published by the American Diabetes Association, 1998.

  The Fitness Book For People with Diabetes. Published by the American Diabetes Association, 1994.

  The "I Hate to Exercise Book" for People with Diabetes by Charlotte Hayes. Published by the American Diabetes Association, 2001.

Fast Food

Americans spend more than $100 billion on fast food every year! Life in the fast lane means that today, more than ever, people with diabetes need to know how to make the best choices at the drive-through window. Fast foods don't totally deserve their "bad guy" reputation. Besides their convenience, portion sizes are standard in each chain from coast to coast, meaning you'll always know their nutrition content from San Diego to St. Augustine. Healthy food choices such as salads, grilled foods, and low-calorie beverages are becoming more common. However, the gigantic portion sizes available also translate into excess sodium and fat, which can sabotage your best eating efforts. The following tips will help you become a better dashboard diner.

- Plan ahead. Think about your choices before you face the fast food menu board. Nutrition information is readily available from most chains. Several pharmaceutical companies have complementary pocket fast food guides you can keep in your car for ready reference. Know the carbohydrate, fat, sodium, and calorie content of your favorites. Determine if they fit into your meal plan.

- Starting your day with a fast food breakfast may get you off on the wrong foot. A breakfast bagel sandwich packs a whopping 690 calories, 59 grams of carbohydrate, 38 grams of fat, and 1560 milligrams of sodium. Choose an English muffin or toast, scrambled egg, Canadian bacon, and low-fat milk instead.
- Downsize, don't super-size. Order small portions (regular, single, or junior), a kid-sized meal, or share the larger servings with your dining companions. A junior bacon cheeseburger rather than the bigger version will save you as much as 200 calories, 11 grams of carbohydrate, 11 grams of fat, and 630 milligrams of sodium.
- Keep high-fat toppings to a minimum. Hold the bacon, cheese, and mayo on the burgers. Keep baked potatoes high in fiber and low in fat by skipping the cheese, butter, sour cream, and bacon.
- A chicken or fish sandwich isn't always a healthier choice than a burger or lean beef sandwich, particularly if the chicken or fish has been breaded and fried.
- Substitute a fresh vegetable salad for french fries or cream-based salads such as potato, macaroni, or pasta. The salad dressing quantity is easier for you to control that way.
- Balance fast food meals with other food choices during the day. If you didn't have a vegetable or fruit at lunch, be sure to add one to your evening menu.

Fat Replacers

Fat replacers are used in reduced-fat foods to give the taste, texture, and appearance of traditional higher-fat foods. Besides being lower in fat, foods with fat replacers are usually, but not always, lower in saturated fat, cholesterol, and calories. Fat replacers can be carbohydrate-based, protein-based, or fat-based. Most reduced-fat and fat-free products contain a mixture of fat replacers.

- **Carbohydrate-based fat replacers** include modified starches, polydextrose, cellulose gum, dextrins, corn syrup solids, maltodextrins, hydrogenated starch hydrolysate, carrageenan, and modified food starch. They work by combining with water to provide a thicker texture, as in fat-free salad dressings. Pureed prunes and applesauce are sometimes used as carbohydrate-based fat replacers in baked goods.

- **Protein-based fat replacers** are protein from egg whites or skim milk. These fat replacers provide a creamy sensation and improve the appearance and texture when fat is removed. They are used in cheese, sour cream, salad dressings, baked goods, butter, and mayonnaise spreads. Simplesse is a protein-based fat replacer primarily found in frozen dairy dessert products.

- **Fat-based replacers** are made from fats that have been altered chemically. Caprenin, olestra, and salatrim are examples of fat-based replacers. They provide few or no calories because the body is unable to fully absorb the fatty acids. They may be used in soft candy, candy coatings, chips, and crackers. These fat replacers may cause cramping and diarrhea and inhibit the absorption of some fat-soluble vitamins.

Most types of fat replacers contribute calories, although less than if fat was used. Fat replacers made from carbohydrate can raise your blood glucose level. How you count fat replacers in your meal plan will depend on what they are made from. Check the Nutrition Facts panel on the food label for calories, carbohydrate, fat, and protein in these foods. If you have questions on how these foods fit into your diabetes meal plan, contact your registered dietitian.

Useful Reference

- **Book**

  A Guide to Fitting Foods with Sugar Substitutes and Fat Replacers Into Your Meal Plan. Published by the American Diabetes Association, 1998.

Fats and Oils

Evidence is clear that fat in the diet is linked to many chronic health problems, with diabetes and heart disease among them. Our bodies do need a small amount of dietary fat (about 15–20% of total calories) to perform a variety of functions. However, most Americans eat far more fat than this. Fats in our diet come from a mixture of different chemicals called fatty acids. These fatty acids act differently on blood lipids, with varying effects on your risk for heart disease and stroke.

- **Monounsaturated fats** are the best fats you can eat because they can lower blood cholesterol. Foods high in monounsaturated fatty acids are liquid at room temperature. Canola, nut, and olive oils are good sources of monounsaturated fat. Replace saturated fat or polyunsaturated fat in your diet with monounsaturated fats.
- **Polyunsaturated fats** can help lower blood cholesterol but at the same time may lower the good cholesterol (HDL) level. Foods high in these fatty acids are liquid or

soft at room temperature. Corn, safflower, soybean, and sunflower oils are high in polyunsaturated fats. Fat in seafood is mainly polyunsaturated, too.

- **Saturated fats** can raise your cholesterol level and increase your risk for heart disease and stroke. People with diabetes should keep their intake of saturated fat to no more than 10% of their total calories. Some individuals (people with LDL cholesterol greater than 100 mg/dl) may benefit from lowering saturated fat intake to less than 7% of energy. Saturated fats come mainly from animal foods, such as meat, poultry, butter, and whole milk and from coconut, palm, and palm kernel oils. Foods high in saturated fatty acids are firm at room temperature. (See *trans fatty acids* below for more information on hydrogenated fats.)
- **Omega-3 fatty acids** are high in a type of polyunsaturated fat. They are mostly found in seafood, especially higher-fat fish, such as albacore tuna, mackerel, and salmon. Soybean and canola oil supply some omega-3 fatty acids also. Research suggests that these fatty acids may help prevent blood platelets from clotting and sticking to artery walls. This may lower the risk for heart attacks. To receive the benefits of omega-3 fatty acids, include two to three servings of fish per week in your meal plan. Although fish oil supplements contain omega-3 fatty acids, they are not advised as a substitute for fish or as a dietary supplement.
- **Trans fatty acids** are formed during the process of hydrogenation. Hydrogenation adds hydrogen molecules to a fatty acid and makes a fat solid when it is at room temperature. Trans fatty acids increase blood cholesterol levels, increasing the risk for heart disease. Most trans fatty acids in the diet come from hydrogenated fats, but they are also found naturally in some foods. Liquid vegetable oil is partially hydrogenated to make some stick margarines. Partially hydrogenated vegetable oil is used in fried foods, baked products, and snack foods.

FAT AND OILS: FOOD SOURCES

Monounsaturated Fats	Polyunsaturated Fats	Saturated Fats	Omega-3 Fatty Acids	Trans Fatty Acids
Avocados	Margarine	Bacon	Albacore tuna	Hydrogenated fats
Olives	Mayonnaise	Butter	Mackerel	Stick margarine
Nuts ▪ Almonds ▪ Peanuts ▪ Pecans ▪ Cashews ▪ Hazelnuts ▪ Pistachios	Corn, safflower, cottonseed, and soybean oil	Coconut and coconut oil	Salmon	Shortening
Olive and canola oil	Walnuts	Cream	Canola and soybean oil	
Sesame seeds	Salad dressing	Cream cheese		
Peanut butter	Pumpkin and sunflower seeds	Shortening		
		Lard		
		Sour cream		
		Palm oil		
		Cocoa butter		
		Meat fat		

It's important to choose sources of fat wisely. Try the tips below to lower your fat intake.

- Choose lean cuts of meat, trim visible fat before cooking, and use preparation methods such as grilling and broiling to decrease fat content.
- Remove skin from poultry and fish.

- Eat fish high in omega-3 fatty acids 2–3 times per week.
- Use low-fat or fat-free milk and other dairy products such as cheese, yogurt, cottage cheese, sour cream, ice cream, and cream cheese.
- Choose soft table spreads instead of stick margarine or butter. Read food labels and select margarine that contains no more than 2 grams of saturated fat per tablespoon and liquid oil as the first ingredient.
- Use vegetable oil instead of solid shortening in cooking and prepare salad dressing or pasta with olive or canola oil.
- Check labels of processed food for palm and coconut oils or other fats. Look for baked products, convenience foods, and snack foods with less than 2 grams of saturated fat per serving.

Useful References

Web Sites

www.nhlbi.nih.gov
www.americanheart.org
www.eatright.org

Books

The Diabetes Carbohydrate and Fat Gram Guide, 2nd Edition by Lea Ann Holzmeister. Published by the American Diabetes Association, 2000.

Diabetes Meal Planning Made Easy: How to Put the Food Pyramid to Work for You, 2nd Edition by Hope Warshaw. Published by the American Diabetes Association, 2000.

Exchange Lists for Meal Planning by the American Diabetes Association and the American Dietetic Association, 1998.

Fiber

The government's *Dietary Guidelines for Americans* recommends that we all include a variety of fiber-containing foods such as whole grains, fruits, and vegetables in our meal plans because they provide vitamins, minerals, fiber, and other substances important for good health. The American Diabetes Association recommends that people with diabetes follow the same advice.

Fiber is not digested and absorbed like other carbohydrates, so it does not affect blood glucose in the same way. Fiber can improve blood fat levels and lower the risk of heart disease, an important consideration for individuals with diabetes. Research in type 2 diabetes has shown that participants eating a high-fiber diet (50 grams per day) had lower glucose, insulin, and blood fat levels than when they ate 24 grams of fiber per day.

Most Americans only eat 8 to 10 grams of fiber daily, so it may be difficult for you to consistently eat the 50 grams of fiber daily that produced positive research study results. Try the following tips to boost your fiber intake.

- Start your day the high-fiber way, with a breakfast cereal with at least 5 grams of fiber per serving.

- Feature beans and grains in your main meal by using them in casseroles, stir-fries, and bean soups. Have a meatless meal once a week.
- Use whole-grain flours, breads, crackers, and noodles.
- Have popcorn, fresh fruit, or raw vegetables for a snack. Keep cleaned, cut-up baby carrots, celery sticks, and fresh fruit ready in your refrigerator for quick snacks.
- When baking, substitute whole-wheat flour for 1/4 to 1/2 of the white flour in a recipe.

If you are using the carbohydrate counting approach to meal planning (see page 34), remember: if there are five or more grams of fiber per serving in a food, subtract them from the total grams of carbohydrate in that serving of food to determine how much carbohydrate is actually available to affect your blood glucose.

First Step in Diabetes Meal Planning

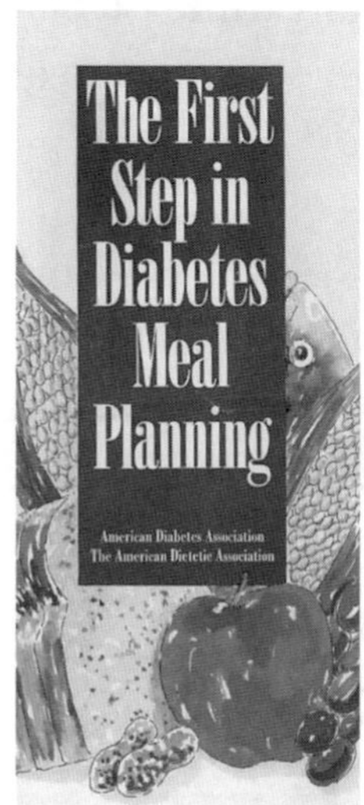

The *First Step in Diabetes Meal Planning* is based on the American Diabetes Association nutrition recommendations for diabetes. It provides self-explanatory, straightforward information about what to eat if you have diabetes. You may find it especially helpful if you are newly diagnosed, or it can provide you with a "refresher course" if you've had diabetes for some time.

The First Step in Diabetes Meal Planning includes goals for healthy eating with diabetes plus a "how to do it" section. It also includes a diabetes food guide pyramid, which uses the exchange list food groupings and daily serving suggestions below.

- **Grains, Beans, and Starchy Vegetables:** 6 or more servings, which could include 1 slice of bread, 4 to 6 crackers, or 1 small potato. These are the base of the pyramid.
- **Vegetables:** 3–5 servings of foods such as 1 cup raw vegetables, 1/2 cup cooked vegetables, or 1/2 cup vegetable juice.

- **Fruits:** 3–4 servings of fruits, which could include 1 small fresh fruit, 1/2 cup canned fruit, 1/4 cup dried fruit, or 1/2 cup fruit juice.
- **Milk:** 2–3 servings, such as 1 cup milk or yogurt.
- **Meat and Others:** 2–3 servings of foods from this group, such as 2–3 ounces cooked lean meat, poultry, or fish; 2–3 ounces of cheese; 1 egg; or 2 tablespoons of peanut butter.
- **Fats, Sweets and Alcohol:** Limit the servings from this group. A serving may include 1 teaspoon of butter or margarine, 1 tablespoon of salad dressing, or 1/2 cup ice cream. These are the tip of the pyramid.

Although this pamphlet is quite self-explanatory, you may find it helpful to review it with a registered dietitian who can tailor it to your specific diabetes goals. You can also use the pamphlet to develop menus or as a checklist to periodically evaluate your eating habits.

Useful References

- **Web Sites**
  www.diabetes.org
  www.eatright.org

Food Diaries

A food diary can help you understand how your eating habits affect your weight and diabetes control. Whether you have type 1 or type 2 diabetes, it can also help you make important decisions about your medication, meal plan, and exercise plan. Research shows that people who keep a food and exercise diary are more successful at weight control than those who don't.

Keeping track of what you eat might clue you into unconscious eating, the portion size your choose, or reasons why you eat. It can be your best strategy for making sense out of your weight, cholesterol, and blood glucose results. If you have just been diagnosed with diabetes, a food diary will give you a picture of your current eating habits and help you and your health care professionals design a realistic meal plan. If you plan to make changes in your schedule, exercise routine, or job, a food diary can help you identify new eating times and amounts. Try the tips below to get started.

- Obtain a notebook or easy-to-use form to record the information. A pocket notebook or even pages in your daily planner can be used. Create your own form on the computer. Be realistic about the size of your record. Make sure you can carry it with you everywhere you go.

- Decide the length of time you will keep your food diary. A two-week food diary examines your eating during weekdays and weekends. A two- to three-day record may be all you can do.
- Record information needed. Keep track of the day, time, food, and portion eaten. You might even keep track of why you ate the food. It may be helpful to keep your blood glucose results and your exercise activities in the same diary. Be specific and honest with yourself about the portion size eaten and the variety or type of food eaten. Regular and fat-free salad dressings contain drastic calorie differences!
- Look up nutrient values of the foods you have eaten. If you are trying to lose weight, you might keep track of calories and fat grams. If you use a carbohydrate counting meal plan, you can record the grams of carbohydrate eaten.
- Use the information you record. Look for patterns in your eating behaviors and blood glucose levels. Identify your problem foods and eating times. Your records may reveal that when you buy bagels you can't resist eating the whole bagel at breakfast, or if candy comes into the house you always overdo it. You might realize it is time for an updated meal plan. If you need help making sense out of your eating habits and the changes needed, bring your diary to your next appointment with your registered dietitian.

Food Labels

Carefully reading food labels will help you make healthy choices for your diabetes meal plan. Today's food labels contain a wealth of information.

- The **nutrition facts panel** gives specific information about the calories, carbohydrate, fat, protein, sodium, fiber, vitamins, and minerals in a single serving of the food. Check out this part of the label to determine if a particular food fits into the carbohydrate guidelines for your meal plan.
- The **ingredient list** lists the ingredients by percentage from most to least. In other words, the product contains the most of the first ingredient and the least of the last ingredient on the list. In this portion of the food label you will find the types of sugars and fats used in the product, such as corn sweeteners or vegetable shortening.
- A **nutrition description** of the product conveys terms such as "low fat" or "high fiber," terms that are carefully defined by government regulations. For example, a "light" food must have 1/3 fewer calories or 50% less fat than the traditional version.

- A **health claim** such as "eating fruits, vegetables, and grain products that contain fiber may help prevent heart disease" is also strictly regulated by the government and must be approved and backed by scientific research before appearing on a product label.

Become familiar with the labels of your favorite foods and read a few new food labels each time you go to the grocery store. Pay particular attention to the following information.

- **Serving size:** Is the serving size noted more or less than the amount you normally eat or the amount specified in your meal plan?
- **Grams of carbohydrate:** Don't focus on the grams of sugar in a product; total carbohydrate is what raises your blood glucose the most. Products labeled "no sugar added" are not necessarily free of carbohydrate. Many foods such as fruits, vegetables, milk, cereals, grains, and legumes have naturally occurring sugars and contain carbohydrate.
- **Grams of fat:** A healthy diet low in fat will help you lose weight and lower your risk for heart disease.

Occasionally your local supermarket may offer a grocery store tour, often led by a registered dietitian, who can help you through the maze of reading food labels. Take advantage of this opportunity to learn more about the foods you typically eat and new items on the market.

Useful Reference

Book

Reading Food Labels: A Handbook for People with Diabetes. Published by the American Diabetes Association and The American Diabetic Association, 1994.

Food Safety

For a person with diabetes, the nausea, vomiting, diarrhea, and inability to eat that accompany foodborne illnesses are not only unpleasant, but may have serious consequences for blood glucose control. The bacteria that cause more than 90% of the cases of foodborne illness can be found everywhere in nature, yet don't affect most individuals unless they find the right conditions: food, moisture, temperature, and time to multiply. To stop bacteria in their tracks, follow the guidelines below.

- Keep food out of "the danger zone" of 40 to 140°F. Don't let any food sit at room temperature longer than two hours. Never thaw foods at room temperature. Use only the refrigerator or microwave for thawing.
- Pay attention to food product "sell by" and "use by" dates in the grocery store. Return home quickly after grocery shopping and store foods properly. Freeze fresh meat, poultry, and seafood immediately if you don't plan to use them within two to three days.
- Wash hands thoroughly with hot soapy water for at least 20 seconds before starting any food preparation. Keep

raw meat, poultry, and seafood and their juices from coming into contact with other foods during preparation. Wash cutting boards with soap and water before preparing any raw food. Never use the same spoon for stirring and tasting a food. Modify recipes that call for uncooked or partially cooked eggs.

- When storing leftovers, divide large amounts into smaller amounts and place them in shallow containers to allow foods to cool more quickly. When reheating leftovers, allow them to become steaming hot or reach a temperature of at least 165°F to destroy any bacteria that may have grown.
- Clean all kitchen surfaces routinely. Launder kitchen towels and dishcloths after one day's use and allow them to dry thoroughly, or use paper towels and throw away after one use. Bacteria can continue to live as long as moisture is available. Experts recommend changing kitchen sponges every two weeks.

If, despite your best precautions, you find yourself the victim of foodborne illness, be sure to follow the diabetes sick day recommendations (see page 212).

Free Foods

They say there's no such thing as a free lunch, but you should be aware that in the world of diabetes nutrition, certain foods don't count! The American Diabetes and American Dietetic Associations define a free food as any food or drink that contains less than 20 calories or less than 5 grams of carbohydrate per serving. Although foods made of pure protein or fat (such as meat, cheese, eggs, peanut butter, oil, and bacon) don't affect blood glucose in the same way that foods containing carbohydrate do, they can be high in calories and should not be considered free foods.

The foods on the following list are examples of those that don't need to be counted in your meal plan, if you limit them to three servings per day, spread throughout the day.

- Fat-free cream cheese: 1 tablespoon
- Powdered nondairy creamer: 2 teaspoons
- Reduced-fat mayonnaise: 1 teaspoon
- Reduced-fat margarine: 1 teaspoon

- Ketchup: 1 tablespoon
- Salsa: 1/4 cup
- Sugar-free syrup: 2 tablespoons

The following list doesn't specify serving sizes and gives examples of things that can be eaten as often as you like.

- Sugar-free gelatin
- Sugar-free chewing gum
- Calorie-free sugar substitutes such as aspartame, saccharin, acesulfame K, or sucralose
- Coffee, tea, and sugar-free beverages
- Seasonings such as herbs, spices, and hot pepper or Worcestershire sauce (you may want to be aware of their sodium content)

Fructosamine Test

Fructosamine is a test similar to the glycohemoglobin test that measures the blood glucose over a period of time. Despite the sound of it, this test has nothing to do with the fructose in food. Fructosamine, which measures the glucose combined with protein in the blood, reflects the level of blood glucose for the past three weeks. It gives different information about your health, and adds a new dimension to our ability to evaluate diabetes.

Individual blood glucose tests are helpful when deciding how you're doing at that very moment, but they do not show the big picture. Glucose levels can change drastically, even in a few minutes. The glycohemoglobin test (see page 124) tells you how your blood glucose control has been over the past few months. The fructosamine test tells you how you've done the past few weeks, so it can detect changes in diabetic control earlier than the glycohemoglobin test.

Fructosamine values are especially useful for short-term follow-up of interventions that have been recently implemented to lower blood glucose. If you have recently started a new medication regimen or eating plan, this test can determine the effectiveness of your changes in two to three weeks. This test should prove very useful for pregnant women with diabetes, who need to know the effect of a treatment change quickly.

Fructosamine tests are not widely used or available, so their place in diabetes care has not been established. Some home meters monitor glucose and fructosamine. As your health care providers become more familiar with its use, more fructosamine tests may be ordered and become available for home use.

Gestational Diabetes Mellitus (GDM)

Gestational diabetes, which is defined as glucose intolerance first recognized during pregnancy, occurs in about 7% of all pregnancies. The majority of cases of gestational diabetes usually disappear once the baby is delivered, but if you have GDM you are at higher risk for developing type 2 diabetes later in life. Good blood glucose control is necessary during your pregnancy to prevent difficulties in labor and delivery and problems in the baby such as macrosomia (when the baby is larger than normal for its age), hypoglycemia, jaundice, and respiratory distress syndrome.

Frequent blood glucose monitoring and a healthy pregnancy meal plan are essential if you have GDM. The American Diabetes Association suggests the following whole blood glucose goals during pregnancy (add 15% to convert the numbers to plasma glucose levels, depending on the glucose meter you use):

- Fasting: 60–90 mg/dl
- Premeal: 60–105 mg/dl
- 1 hour after meals: 100–120 mg/dl
- 2–6 hours after meals: 60–120 mg/dl

If your blood glucose levels remain out of the target range, insulin therapy may be necessary, although some physicians do recommend certain oral diabetes medicines during pregnancy. Excellent blood glucose control is the goal, no matter what approach is used.

Nutrition for pregnancy with GDM should focus on good nutrition for the baby, with an appropriate weight gain, normal blood glucose, and prevention of urinary ketones for you. The amount of weight you should gain during pregnancy depends on your weight before you got pregnant. In general, a woman of normal weight should gain 25–35 pounds during her pregnancy. You may be advised by your health care team to gain less if you were previously overweight, or more if you were underweight. Your rate of weight gain should be quite small during the first trimester, but will increase later as your pregnancy progresses.

You should work with a registered dietitian to design an individualized meal plan that is consistent in carbohydrate, because carbohydrate is the nutrient that has the most immediate impact on blood glucose levels. The nutrition and medical recommendations you receive will be based on your glucose response to certain foods and their effects at different times of day. Interestingly, most women with GDM need to limit their carbohydrate at breakfast to 15–30 grams because of hormones that interfere with the action of insulin.

Of course, adjustments to your meal plan should be made based on your blood glucose monitoring results. In most cases, your nutrition plan should provide three meals a day, with two to four between-meal snacks. An evening snack is particularly important to prevent hypoglycemia during the night and urinary ketones in the morning. Urinary ketones are a sign of starvation, which increases risk of complications to the baby. An evening snack can provide the nutrition you and your baby need through the night.

As with any pregnancy, a well-balanced diet with about 60 grams of protein will provide you with the vitamins and minerals you need; however, prenatal vitamins and minerals are often recommended as nutritional "insurance." At this time, research shows that the four most common sugar substitutes (acesulfame K, aspartame, saccharin, and sucralose) are safe to use during pregnancy in moderation. (Saccharin does cross the placenta and can reach the baby, but there is no evidence that it causes ill effects.) Discuss your use of sugar substitutes with your health care team.

Other dietary considerations include alcohol (which should be avoided because it can cause birth defects) and caffeine (a stimulant that you may need to avoid during pregnancy.) Pregnant women should avoid raw fish to reduce the risk of viral and bacterial illness. Recent research also suggests that pregnant women and nursing mothers should not eat shark, swordfish, king mackerel, and tilefish because the methyl mercury they contain may harm the unborn baby's developing nervous system.

Managing gestational diabetes means paying extra attention to your lifestyle during this important time. The commitment you make now will pay off with the best pregnancy outcome—a healthy, happy baby! For more information about pregnancy if you already have type 1 or type 2 diabetes, see page 196.

Useful Reference

- **Book**

  Gestational Diabetes: What to Expect, 4th Edition. Published by the American Diabetes Association, 2000.

Glucagon

Glucagon is a hormone made in the alpha cells of the pancreas that raises glucose and can be injected in severe hypoglycemia. In severe hypoglycemia, your brain has inadequate amounts of glucose, and you can lose consciousness or become uncooperative. If you are elderly and taking oral diabetes medications or insulin, you are at especially high risk for developing severe hypoglycemia.

Glucagon emergency kits include a syringe with 1 milligram of glucagon, one of the major hormones that raise glucose. The injection of glucagon raises your blood glucose so that you regain consciousness within 20 minutes. Glucagon corrects your severe hypoglycemia for about an hour after you receive the injection. As soon as you are able to swallow, you should have some carbohydrate liquid such as juice, soda, or low-fat milk. You should then eat a substantial snack containing carbohydrate and protein such as a half sandwich or cheese and crackers to restore glycogen stores in the liver and to keep your blood glucose levels from falling before the next meal.

Monitor your blood glucose frequently for several hours after a glucagon injection to detect further episodes of hypoglycemia and also hyperglycemia due to overtreatment. Remember to contact your health care provider about your episode of severe hypoglycemia in case your diabetes treatment plan needs adjustment.

Talk with your health care professionals about whether you should buy a glucagon emergency kit, which is available by prescription. The kit has a special glucagon syringe that is filled with a diluting solution. Keep glucagon with you at all times. Read the instructions that come with the kit and teach family, friends, coworkers, and school personnel how to use it.

Useful References

- **Web Site**
  www.diabetes.org

- **Books**
  101 Tips for Staying Healthy with Diabetes (& Avoiding Complications), 2nd Edition by David Schade. Published by the American Diabetes Association, 1999.

  The Uncomplicated Guide to Diabetes Complications by Marvin E. Levin and Michael Pfeifer. Published by the American Diabetes Association, 1998.

Glucose Intolerance

Glucose intolerance refers to the stage between normal blood glucose levels and diabetes (high blood glucose levels). It is considered a risk factor for the development of diabetes and heart disease. Glucose intolerance can be divided into two classifications.

- **Impaired Fasting Glucose (IFG):** The plasma glucose level after an 8-hour fast is greater than 110 mg/dl but less than 126 mg/dl. It's thought that about 7% of the U.S. population has IFG.
- **Impaired Glucose Tolerance (IGT):** IGT occurs when the plasma glucose level at the 2-hour point of an oral glucose tolerance test is between 140 to 199 mg/dl. Almost 11% of American adults have IGT.

Both IFG and IGT are associated with insulin resistance, which may precede the onset of type 2 diabetes. Insulin resistance is a factor in Syndrome X (a condition where heart disease risk factors such as high blood pressure, high blood fats, and high blood glucose are clustered together) and polycystic ovary disease, a common cause of female infertility. Most people with type 2 diabetes have some form of insulin resistance, in which the body is unable to use insulin efficiently, resulting in an elevated blood glucose level with a higher than normal amount of insulin produced by the pancreas.

If you have glucose intolerance, you should not dismiss it as "just a touch of sugar." Follow up on nutrition concerns to prevent diabetes and heart disease. Work on your weight through calorie control and increasing physical activity. Take steps such as the DASH diet (see page 60) to prevent high blood pressure and limit the fat in your diet to improve abnormal blood fat levels.

Glycemic Index

The glycemic index (GI) is a meal-planning tool for diabetes that ranks foods containing carbohydrate according to their potential to raise blood glucose levels. Pure glucose, which evokes the greatest blood glucose response, has a glycemic index of 100. Other foods are ranked according to how most people react after eating them, in comparison to their response to pure glucose. To standardize the results, each serving of test food contains 50 grams of carbohydrate. More than 600 foods have been tested and assigned a glycemic index number. Glycemic index numbers range from low (red kidney beans, GI of 27) to intermediate (canned sweet corn, GI of 55) to high (instant mashed potatoes, GI of 86).

In general, carbohydrate foods that break down quickly during digestion, such as most flaked breakfast cereals, have the highest glycemic index values. Carbohydrates that break down slowly, such as most fiber-rich breakfast cereals, release glucose gradually into the bloodstream and have lower glycemic index values. Other key factors influencing the glycemic index of a food are the amount of fat it contains, the type of starch it's composed of, the physical form of the food, its fiber content, and the cooking and processing methods used during its preparation.

This method of meal planning has been used for more than 20 years, particularly in Europe and Australia, and continues to be extensively tested and refined. However, it is not wise to base your food selections solely on glycemic index information. For example, potato chips and french fries have a lower glycemic index than a baked potato, but you should consider their fat content as well as their effect on blood glucose. Many foods containing refined sugar have a moderate glycemic index, but their empty calories still mean that they shouldn't become a major part of your diet. The complexity of the glycemic index makes it a challenge to put into practice. The current Nutrition Recommendations of the American Diabetes Association do not endorse its use, preferring instead to emphasize the total amount, rather than the source, of carbohydrate in the meal plan.

Useful Reference

- **Book**

  The Glucose Revolution—The Authoritative Guide to the Glycemic Index. Jennie Brand-Miller, Thomas Wolever, Stephen Colagiuri, and Kaye Foster-Powell. Published by Marlowe & Company, New York, 1999.

Glycohemoglobin Test

A blood test called a glycohemoglobin (HbA_{1c}) test can give you an overall picture of how well your diabetes management plan is working and whether changes are needed. This blood test measures the glucose attached to hemoglobin in red blood cells. Hemoglobin carries oxygen from the lungs to all the cells of the body. The more glucose in your blood, the more red blood cells have glucose attached to their hemoglobin, and the higher your glycohemoglobin test results.

This test tells you your average blood glucose level for the past two to four months. Your glucose control over a period of time is just as important as control throughout each day. Individual blood glucose checks tell you how you're doing at the moment, but they do not give the big picture. Blood glucose levels can change in less than an hour. For example, you may check your glucose levels before meals and find they are in the normal range, yet your glycohemoglobin results are elevated. This may be because your blood glucose levels are high two hours after a meal.

It is important to use your home blood glucose readings and glycohemoglobin results together when evaluating your diabetes control. If your average blood glucose level is high, something in your plan may need to be changed.

If your blood glucose control improves, it takes about three to four months to see the results in an HbA_{1c} test. Testing more frequently is usually not done, except in special situations such as pregnancy when tight blood glucose control is essential. When you are diagnosed with diabetes, a glycohemoglobin test should be done. After that, the American Diabetes Association recommends that people using insulin have a glycohemoglobin test done at least four times a year. If you don't use insulin, have the test done as your doctor recommends. Your health care providers may also have the test done when there has been a change in treatment. This helps evaluate the effectiveness of the treatment change.

There are several types of glycohemoglobin tests. Common ones are the HbA_{1c} and the HbA_1. Different tests and different labs have different "normal ranges." If you change doctors or laboratories, find out what numbers from your new laboratory mean. Find out the type of test and your results. Research has shown that keeping glycohemoglobin at 7% or under decreases diabetes complications. Discuss your glycohemoglobin goal with your health care providers.

Goal Setting

Taking care of your diabetes involves knowledge, time, resources, support, and the desire to stay healthy. There may be aspects of your diabetes management that you have had difficulty implementing or improvements in your health that you desire. Maybe you would like to lose weight and improve your blood glucose control. It might be that your health care providers have suggested a change in your medication and you are reluctant. Making improvements in your health and diabetes control means setting goals and a plan for achieving those goals.

Discuss your goals with your health care providers and listen as they explore goals they might have for you. To set effective goals, you need to understand why they are necessary and want to make the change. If your registered dietitian recommends a change in your meal plan and you are unable to meet this goal, your management plan will not be successful. Mutually agreed-upon goals improve your chances of success.

Before setting behavior or lifestyle goals, it is important to establish your health and diabetes management goals. Discuss your blood glucose targets, blood lipid goals, and weight goals with your health care providers. Explore your desire to prevent diabetes complications and maintain good health. Establishing your interest in good diabetes control and overall good health will clarify your motivation and desire to make behavior changes.

Behavior change goals are the "what to do" part of goal setting. For example, to help you lose five pounds you may set a goal of keeping a food record for five days during the next two weeks. Sometimes your health care provider will have you write these goals down to help you remember and commit yourself to the plan. Remember to set realistic goals that allow a reasonable time frame for the change to happen. Losing five pounds in one week is not realistic or healthy.

It may help to set short-term and long-term goals. A long-term goal is your intention over a period of time, such as "I will lose 20 pounds in the next year." Break your long-term goal into more realistic small actions or the "how to do it" part of goal setting. A short-term goal might specify the healthy eating habits you will adopt to reach your long-term goal. For example, you will reduce your daily calorie intake by substituting lower-calorie snacks and exercising three times a week.

Part of goal setting is to evaluate your success or progress of your goals. Think about how you benefited from the lifestyle changes. Review your diabetes control and health status with your health care providers. You might even want to establish a personal non-food reward for making lifestyle changes. This may help motivate you to set additional goals. Special time with family or friends, a fun shopping trip, or a mini vacation are common rewards.

At each visit with your health care provider, evaluate your goals and establish new goals to improve your health and diabetes control.

Gram

A gram is a unit of weight in the metric system. One pound equals 454 grams and one ounce equals about 28 grams.

Carbohydrate is also measured in grams (g), but don't confuse this with the gram weight of a food. One slice of bread may weigh 30 grams, but contains only 15 grams of carbohydrate. An 1800-calorie diet may contain 225 grams of carbohydrate. If you use the carbohydrate counting meal-planning method, you will keep track of the number of grams of carbohydrate you eat at meals and snacks.

Grocery Shopping

What you purchase at supermarkets and bring home has a great deal to do with what you and your family eat. With thousands of foods offered at the supermarkets, careful shopping habits and a commitment to healthy eating are essential to successful diabetes meal planning. Follow the tips below for greater grocery store success.

- **Go to the market with a plan.** Refer to your diabetes meal plan and the diabetes food guide pyramid when selecting foods and planning shopping lists and menus. The foods at the base of the pyramid should fill the largest space in your cart.
- **Plan your menus before you shop.** This gives you ideas for making shopping and preparation faster and easier. Plan meals for several days to help you meet your eating goals.
- **Keep a shopping list and stick to it.** Refer to your menus when developing your list and write down foods as you run out. Keep healthy foods on hand to make cooking quick and healthy. Write down the amount to

purchase as indicated in recipes or menus. Organize your list by category to match the store layout. This saves time and helps you avoid those supermarket traps. Stick to your list to avoid impulse buying. Impulse buying can drive your food budget out of control and your meal plan to disaster.

- **Check for specials.** When possible and nutritionally sound, plan your menus and purchases around weekly specials or availability of coupons. Buy fruits and vegetables in season for tasty savings.
- **Look for fresh, safe, and high-quality food.** Look for use-before/sell-by/ best-if-used-by dates to tell you the quality and safety of foods. Produce, meat, poultry, fish, deli foods, and dairy foods should appear fresh. The store should be clean and neat.
- **Use nutrition labels to guide your choices.** Reading food labels helps you determine whether the food is nutritionally sound, works with your health goals, and contains the nutrients you want. Understand the Nutrition Facts section, health claims, ingredient panels, and nutrition descriptors.

Useful References

Books

Complete Guide to Convenience Food Counts by Lea Ann Holzmeister. Published by the American Diabetes Association, 2001.

Diabetes Meal Planning on $7 a Day or Less by Patti B. Geil and Tami A. Ross. Published by the American Diabetes Association, 1999.

Healthy Food Choices

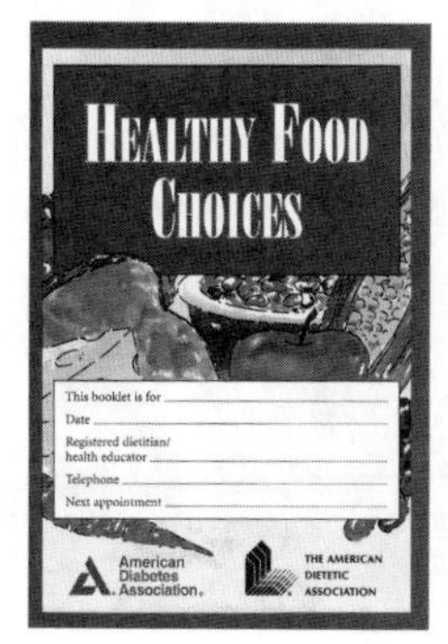

Healthy Food Choices is a two-part pamphlet that can help you learn more about healthy eating practices. It provides straightforward information about the basics of healthy eating, weight loss, carbohydrate counting, and simplified exchange meal planning. *Healthy Food Choices* provides you with basic diabetes nutrition advice, such as:

- Eat a variety of foods.
- Avoid skipping meals.
- Eat healthy carbohydrates.
- Watch serving sizes.
- Eat less fat.
- Maintain a healthy weight.
- Be physically active.

This pamphlet also folds open to include space for you to identify your personal health goals and choose the steps you can take to achieve them. A registered dietitian can review *Healthy Food Choices* with you to personalize it for your diabetes treatment plan. Although this approach provides useful information, you may want a more structured way to plan your meals such as *Exchange Lists for Meal Planning* (see page 86) or *Carbohydrate Counting* (see page 34).

Useful References

- **Web Sites**
  www.diabetes.org
  www.eatright.org

Heart Disease

People with diabetes are at increased risk for atherosclerosis or heart disease. Atherosclerosis is hardening of the arteries. Large blood vessels become narrowed or blocked by a buildup of plaque. Plaque is made from fats and cholesterol. When blood cholesterol and fat levels are too high, this can cause plaque to accumulate in the inner walls of blood vessels. Clogged and narrowed blood vessels make it harder for enough healthy blood to get to all parts of your body. This can cause many serious problems.

When arteries become clogged and narrowed, you may have one or more of the heart problems below.

- **Chest pain,** also called angina.
- **Heart attack.** A heart attack happens when a blood vessel in or near the heart becomes blocked. Not enough blood can get to that part of the heart muscle. That area of the heart muscle stops working, so the heart is weaker. During a heart attack, you may have chest pain along with nausea, indigestion, extreme weakness, and sweating.

Clogged arteries can also cause lack of blood flow to the brain, which is called a stroke. Symptoms of a stroke are sudden weakness; numbness of your face, arm, or leg on one side of your body; sudden confusion; trouble talking; dizziness; and vision problems.

Decreased blood flow to the legs and feet can cause peripheral vascular disease. You may feel pain in your buttocks, the back of your legs, or your thighs when you stand, walk, or exercise. Other signs of peripheral vascular disease are cold feet, loss of hair on the feet or on the knuckles of the hand, shiny feet, and thickened toenails.

The following factors contribute to heart disease:

- High blood sugar.
- High blood pressure.
- Cigarette smoking.
- High blood cholesterol and other abnormal blood fat levels.
- A diet high in saturated fat and cholesterol.
- Being overweight.
- Inactivity.

To reduce your risk of heart disease:

- Stop smoking.
- Control your weight.
- Control your blood sugar and blood pressure.
- Lower your blood fat levels.
- Take your diabetes, blood pressure, and heart medications faithfully.
- Exercise regularly.

- Follow the healthy eating plan you work out with your registered dietitian.
- Get regular medical checkups and tell your health care provider if you have any of the symptoms mentioned above.

Useful References

Web Sites

www.niddk.nih.gov
www.americanheart.org

Book

The Uncomplicated Guide to Diabetes Complications by Marvin E. Levin and Michael A. Pfeifer. Published by the American Diabetes Association, 1998.

Herbals and Supplements

More than 40% of Americans use herbals and other dietary supplements, yet less than half of them share this information with their health care providers. In 1994, the Dietary Supplement and Health Education Act (DSHEA) was passed by Congress. This legislation moved herbals and other similar products into the category of "dietary supplements," exempting them from the same stringent approval process that is required for drugs. This means that herbals and supplements do not require proof that they are safe and effective to be marketed. Since individuals with diabetes often take a number of other medications, they should be especially cautious when using dietary supplements because of the potential for serious side effects and drug interactions.

Until more carefully designed human studies can be completed on these products, it's important to be cautious. The safety and effectiveness of these supplements are largely unproven. Before taking any supplement, be sure to read and follow the tips below.

- Keep your health care team informed about any dietary supplements you may be taking. These products may have side effects and interact with other medical conditions, drugs, nutrients, or therapies.

- Supplements should only be used in addition to, and not as replacements for, the essential elements of your diabetes care regimen, such as meal planning, physical activity, and medications.
- Remember that "natural" does not necessarily mean "safe." Because most supplements are not subject to rigorous government safety and efficacy testing, they may be potentially more dangerous than conventional forms of medication.
- Do not use herbals or supplements if you are pregnant or breastfeeding. The effects of these products on the baby are unknown. Do not give children herbal supplements without first consulting your pediatrician.
- Do background research on a product before you begin taking it, particularly since many products are very expensive and may provide only questionable health benefits.
- Read labels carefully and look for telephone numbers, addresses, and web sites on the labels of products so you can ask questions of the manufacturers. Beware of products containing only testimonials instead of proven research results. Also, the "active" ingredient in a herbal or supplement is often not standard from product to product. Purchase products that are standardized from companies that meet "Good Manufacturing Practice" (GMP) guidelines, as noted on the product label, to ensure product purity and safety.
- If you choose to use a dietary supplement, it is usually better to start with single-ingredient products rather than multiple-ingredient products because if you experience an adverse effect or a worsening of blood glucose it would be difficult to determine which ingredient is responsible. Begin with a small dose of a prod-

uct and work up to the recommended dose to determine whether the supplement has any effect on blood glucose levels. For some products, it may take several weeks to determine whether there is any effect on blood glucose.

- Monitor your blood glucose levels frequently when taking any type of nutritional supplement and share any concerns about changes in blood glucose with your health care team. Remember—taking a pill will not make up for an unhealthy lifestyle.
- Make careful note of any symptoms such as headaches, nausea, or rash that may be side effects from a supplement. If symptoms persist, stop taking the supplement and see your health care team.

Useful References

Web Sites

www.alternativediabetes.com
www.nal.usda.gov/fnic/IBIDS
www.naturaldatabase.com

Books

The Health Professional's Guide to Popular Dietary Supplements by Allison Sarubin. Published by The American Dietetic Association, 2000.

Tyler's Honest Herbal by Steven Foster and Varro E. Tyler. Published by The Haworth Herbal Press, 2000.

Honeymoon Phase

The honeymoon phase is the time period, usually less than a year, after the initial diagnosis of type 1 diabetes when the need for injections of insulin is reduced or eliminated. Beta cells in the pancreas continue to function by still releasing insulin. This period lasts longer when diabetes is diagnosed at an older age, the initial presentation of the disease is milder, and the amount of islet cell antibodies is lower. The honeymoon phase ends with a sudden or slowly increasing requirement for insulin.

Keeping blood glucose levels close to the normal range is much easier during this phase. Insulin doses are decreased and the number of injections required may also decrease. Frequent blood glucose monitoring continues to be important to detect blood glucose changes and the need for treatment changes. Maintaining a diabetes meal plan during the honeymoon period establishes eating habits that will be essential when the phase is over. Food intake amounts may be more flexible since some insulin is available from the pancreas.

Useful References

Web Sites

www.childrenwithdiabetes.com
www.diabetes123.com
www.diabetes.org

Hyperglycemia

Too much glucose in the blood is known as hyperglycemia (blood glucose of 140 mg/dl or above). Symptoms of hyperglycemia include headache, blurry vision, excessive thirst and hunger, fatigue, frequent urination, upset stomach, and fruity smell on the breath (if diabetic ketoacidosis is present). Hyperglycemia over the long term can damage your eyes, kidneys, heart, nerves, and blood vessels. Blood glucose levels can also be high for a short time and cause a life-threatening situation known as diabetic ketoacidosis that could result in coma or death. Hyperglycemia may have more subtle symptoms than hypoglycemia, so regularly testing your blood glucose is vitally important if you have diabetes.

Hyperglycemia can be caused by a variety of factors including eating too much food or carbohydrate, skipping or taking too little medication, stress, illness, infection, or skipping your usual exercise or physical activity. There are other reasons blood glucose can be elevated as well. The **dawn phenomenon** refers to the body's normal mechanism that allows blood glucose to rise between 4 and 8 a.m. to wake you up and give you energy for the day. If you wake up with mysteriously high morning blood glucose levels, your diabetes team may suggest a change in your meal plan or medication to treat this situation.

Another reason for hyperglycemia may be the **Somogyi effect**. Ironically, this elevation in morning blood glucose occurs due to a "rebound" of blood glucose in the morning, after having hypoglycemia or low blood glucose between 2 and 4 a.m. If your diabetes team suspects you are experiencing the Somogyi effect, they may recommend that you set your alarm to test your blood glucose between 2 and 4 a.m. A change in your insulin may be needed.

Finally, people with type 2 diabetes can experience a condition called **hyperglycemic hyperosmolar nonketotic syndrome (HHNS)**, which severely elevates blood glucose to levels over 600 mg/dl, requiring immediate medical treatment. HHNS occurs most often in the elderly and individuals with restricted mobility. Again, frequent blood glucose testing is the best way to prevent these situations.

The American Diabetes Association recommends the following treatment approaches for hyperglycemia.

If your blood glucose is between 180 and 250 mg/dl, your physician may tell you to try one of the following:

- a small extra dose of short-acting insulin;
- a walk or some other exercise or physical activity;
- reducing the amount of food in your next meal or snack.

If your blood glucose stays above 250 mg/dl:

- check for signs of diabetic ketoacidosis or HHNS and call your doctor immediately if you have symptoms.

If your blood glucose stays above 350 mg/dl:

- call your doctor.

If your blood glucose stays above 500 mg/dl:

- call your doctor and have someone take you to a hospital emergency room immediately.

Useful References

Books

American Diabetes Association Complete Guide to Diabetes, 2nd Edition. Published by The American Diabetes Association, 1999.

Diabetes A to Z, 4th Edition. Published by The American Diabetes Association, 2000.

Hypertension

Hypertension, or high blood pressure, is a dangerous condition that occurs when the heart is working harder than it should. Six out of ten people with diabetes have hypertension (blood pressure greater than or equal to 140/90 mmHg), and controlling it will reduce the rate of progression of diabetes complications such as nephropathy (diabetes kidney complications) and heart disease. The American Diabetes Association suggests that adults with diabetes maintain their blood pressure at less than 130/80 mmHg. Changes in lifestyle are the first steps to keeping blood pressure under control. Weight loss, reducing the amount of sodium in the diet, and limiting alcoholic beverages are all steps you should try before beginning medications.

- **Weight loss.** Excess body weight is closely related to high blood pressure, particularly if excess fat is deposited on the upper part of the body ("apple-shaped"). Blood pressure will improve with a weight loss of as little as 10 pounds.
- **Sodium.** The sodium found in sodium chloride (table salt) is positively linked to levels of blood pressure—

that is, the higher your intake of sodium, the higher your blood pressure level. This is particularly true in people who are sodium sensitive, such as African Americans, older people, and people with diabetes. For people with mild to moderate hypertension, less than 2400 mg/day of sodium is recommended. The vast majority of sodium in our diets is found in processed foods, convenience foods, and salty snack foods. One teaspoon of table salt contains 2400 mg of sodium.

- **Alcoholic beverages.** Too much alcohol is a risk factor for high blood pressure and stroke and may interfere with the effectiveness of blood pressure-lowering medication. Limit your daily alcohol intake to less than two drinks daily if you are a man and to no more than one drink daily if you are a woman. A drink is defined as 12 ounces of beer, 5 ounces of wine, or 1 1/2 ounces of 80-proof distilled spirits.

The most successful nutrition approach to improving your blood pressure is the DASH (Dietary Approaches to Stop Hypertension) eating plan, which is described more fully on page 60. Speak with your physician and registered dietitian about an individualized plan to prevent or control your hypertension.

Useful Reference

- **Web Site**
  www.nih.gov/health/hbp-tifl

Hypoglycemia

Hypoglycemia occurs when blood glucose levels get too low, usually below 70 mg/dl. Symptoms of hypoglycemia include shakiness, confusion, sweatiness, irritability, fatigue, hunger, and personality change. If untreated, hypoglycemia can lead to seizures or loss of consciousness. It can occur in people with diabetes who take insulin injections or certain oral diabetes medicines that stimulate insulin production such as sulfonylureas, thiazolidinediones, meglitinides, and D-phenylalanine derivatives.

Hypoglycemia usually occurs just before meals, during or after strenuous exercise, or when insulin is acting at its peak. Some individuals with diabetes, particularly pregnant women and those with tightly controlled blood glucose, lose the ability to recognize the warning symptoms of low blood glucose until their blood glucose level has fallen to a dangerous level. If you think you may have hypoglycemic unawareness, talk with your diabetes team. They may recommend that you increase the number of times you test your blood glucose daily, suggest that you always test your blood glucose before driving, and advise you to educate the people around you about the symptoms and treatment of hypoglycemia.

Hypoglycemia can be caused by a number of factors, including eating too little food or carbohydrate, delaying or skipping a meal or snack, exercising harder or longer or being more physically active than usual, taking too much insulin or diabetes medication, illness, or drinking alcohol on an empty stomach. If you think you are experiencing hypoglycemia, immediate treatment is essential. You should check your blood glucose level if possible and follow the treatment approaches recommended by the American Diabetes Association for hypoglycemia.

If your blood glucose is under 70 mg/dl:

- eat or drink something with about 15 grams of carbohydrate;
- wait 15 to 20 minutes, then check again.

If your blood glucose is still below 70 mg/dl:

- eat or drink something with about 15 grams of carbohydrate;
- wait 15–20 minutes, then check again;

If your blood glucose is still below 70 mg/dl, call your doctor or have someone take you to a hospital emergency room immediately.

If your blood glucose is over 70 mg/dl:

- stop eating or drinking carbohydrate foods, even though you may still feel the symptoms of hypoglycemia (more carbohydrate than you need can result in high blood glucose for the remainder of the day).

If your next meal is more than an hour away:

- eat a small snack of carbohydrate and protein, such as a slice of low-fat cheese with crackers.

You may experience severe hypoglycemia and be unable to treat it yourself. It's best to take precautions ahead of time to prevent this from happening. Always be alert to your symptoms of hypoglycemia and treat yourself immediately. For people with type 1 diabetes, it's also a good idea to have a glucagon emergency kit and educate the people around you in its use. (See page 118 for more information).

When blood glucose levels are 50–60 mg/dl, 15 grams of carbohydrate can be expected to raise blood glucose levels about 50 mg/dl over 40–45 minutes. The following foods each contain about 10–15 grams of carbohydrate and can be used to treat hypoglycemia.

Glucose tablets or gel (check dosage on package)

4 ounces fruit juice or regular soft drink

6–8 ounces fat-free or low-fat milk

2 tablespoons raisins

3–4 teaspoons sugar

5–7 Lifesavers

1 tablespoon honey or corn syrup

Useful References

Books

American Diabetes Association Complete Guide to Diabetes, 2nd Edition. Published by The American Diabetes Association, 1999.

Diabetes A to Z, 4th Edition. Published by The American Diabetes Association, 2000.

Insulin

Insulin is a hormone that helps the body use glucose for energy. The beta cells of the pancreas make insulin. When the body cannot make enough insulin on its own, a person with diabetes must inject insulin made from other sources, either animal insulin (pork or pork/beef) or human insulin made with bacteria in a laboratory. Insulin lowers blood glucose by moving glucose from the blood into the cells of your body. Once inside the cells, glucose provides energy. Insulin lowers your blood glucose whether you eat or not. You should eat on time if you take insulin to avoid hypoglycemia.

If you have type 1 diabetes, your pancreas no longer make insulin and you must take insulin shots. If you have type 2 diabetes, your pancreas may not make enough insulin or your body has a hard time using your insulin. You may need to take diabetes medicines and/or you may need to take insulin.

There are several types of insulin. They each work at different speeds. People respond differently to different types of insulin, so it is important to find the type of insulin that works best for you. Many people take two types of insulin.

INSULIN ACTION

Insulin Type	Starts working (Onset) (hours)	Lowers blood glucose most (Peak) (hours)	Finishes working (Duration) (hours)
Rapid Acting			
• Human lispro	Within 15 minutes	1–1 1/2	4–5
Short Acting			
• Human regular	1/2–1	2–3	4–6
Intermediate Acting			
• Human NPH	2–4	4–10	10–16
• Human Lente	3–4	4–12	12–18
Long Acting			
• Human Ultralente	6–10	14–24	18–20
• Glargine	4–6	no peak	24

Insulin is available in a combination of rapid acting, short acting, and intermediate acting. You can mix them yourself or buy the insulin premixed in a specific ratio. Mixtures of regular and NPH insulin come in combinations of 50/50 and 70/30. This means that the mixture contains 50 or 70% NPH and 50 or 30% regular insulin. 75/25 insulin contains 75% NPL insulin (a variation of NPH) and 25% lispro insulin. Premixed insulins are useful for people with busy schedules or people with eyesight or dexterity problems. If you take premixed insulin, make sure you understand what type of insulin you will be taking and how it affects your blood glucose levels.

Follow the tips below to store your insulin.

- Unopened bottles can be stored in the refrigerator and must be discarded after the date on the bottle.
- Opened bottles of insulin can be stored in the refrigerator and must be discarded after three months.

- Opened bottles kept at room temperature must be discarded after one month.
- If insulin gets too hot or cold, it breaks down and does not work. So, do not keep insulin in very cold places such as the freezer, or in hot places, such as by a window or in the car's glove compartment during warm weather.
- Regular, lispro, or glargine insulin should be clear, with no floating pieces or color.
- NPH, Lente, or Ultralente insulin should be cloudy, without floating pieces or crystals.

The goal of insulin therapy is to keep blood glucose levels as close to normal at all times. The best insulin therapy plan for you will depend on how easy it is to control your blood glucose levels and how well you understand how food, physical activity, and stress affect your diabetes.

Insulin Pump Therapy

An insulin pump is a small battery-powered mechanical device, a little larger than a deck of cards, which delivers insulin into the body. The pump is worn outside the body in a pouch or on a belt holder. It connects to a narrow, flexible tubing that ends with a needle inserted just under the skin near the abdomen. Many people with diabetes like insulin pumps because they provide convenience, flexibility, and improved blood glucose control. The insulin pump can smooth out blood glucose swings and take care of nighttime lows and morning highs.

Pumps deliver insulin in two different ways, the basal rate and a pre-meal bolus. Users set the pump to give a steady trickle or "basal" amount of insulin continuously throughout the day. Most pumps today have the option for setting several basal rates. Pumps release "bolus" doses of insulin (several units at a time) at meals and at times when blood glucose is too high based on the users' programming. Frequent blood glucose monitoring is essential to determine insulin dosages and to ensure that insulin is delivered.

Pre-meal boluses are designed to cover the food you eat during a meal. Since you can program the bolus any time, you have much greater flexibility with regard to mealtime and contents. If you decide to eat late, you just program the bolus later than usual.

You must program the pump to deliver insulin when you want it. And you must still monitor your blood sugar, many times a day. Wearing an insulin pump will probably require more work on your part than traditional injection therapy.

People who successfully use an insulin pump are dedicated in the management of their diabetes. They understand the way in which food, exercise, and insulin work together to raise and lower blood glucose levels. Carbohydrate counting is a great tool for achieving blood glucose control when using an insulin pump. It gives you a method to match your pre-meal bolus dose of insulin to the actual amount of food you plan to eat. (See page 34 for more information on carbohydrate counting.)

Intensive Insulin Therapy

Intensive diabetes therapy is a form of treatment where the main objective is to keep blood glucose levels as close to the normal range as possible to prevent diabetes complications. Two well-known studies, the DCCT and the UKPDS, demonstrated that diabetes complications decreased by keeping blood glucose levels as close to normal as possible. (See pages 64 and 240 for more information on these studies.)

For people with type 1 diabetes, intensive insulin therapy usually refers to three or more insulin shots a day or use of an insulin pump, testing blood glucose levels four to seven times each day, and adjusting insulin doses to match exercise and food intake. For people with type 2 diabetes, the methods of therapy used for reaching blood glucose goals can be quite different, and a trial and error approach may be used. Meeting your goals might require a combination approach of two oral diabetes medications or oral medications and insulin.

Intensive therapy aims to keep your blood glucose levels very close to normal. With this goal, there may be some risks. Because you are keeping your blood glucose levels lower, your chances of having low blood glucose reactions are greater, and you may also gain some weight. Intensive management for both type 1 and type 2 diabetes requires additional education and frequent office or phone visits with your health care team.

Following an individual meal plan is an important part of intensive management for type 1 and type 2 diabetes. In fact, your food choices may be more flexible when you use intensive diabetes management. If you take insulin, you may be able to eat to your preferences and schedule and adjust your insulin accordingly. With intensive therapy you can adjust your rapid- or short-acting insulin to cover the carbohydrate content of your meals and snacks. The carbohydrate-to-insulin ratio is an advanced method of meal planning used with intensive insulin therapy. In this approach you calculate your insulin dose based on your carbohydrate intake and blood glucose results.

Your registered dietitian will help you through the meal planning steps below before you begin intensive insulin therapy.

- Establish a consistent eating pattern.
- Implement a successful insulin regimen for your usual eating pattern.
- Identify food portions and carbohydrate content.
- Monitor your blood glucose four to five times every day.

Individuals who are good candidates for intensive management include healthy adults with type 1 or type 2 diabetes, certain adolescents and older children, women with diabetes who are pregnant or who plan a pregnancy, and patients who have had or will have kidney transplantation for diabetic nephropathy. Check with your health care professionals about your blood glucose goals and your interest in intensive management.

Useful References

- **Web Site**
  www.diabetes.org

- **Books**
  American Diabetes Association Complete Guide to Diabetes, 2nd Edition. Published by the American Diabetes Association, 1999.

  Diabetes A to Z, 4th Edition. Published by the American Diabetes Association, 2000.

Internet Nutrition Advice

The Internet can serve as a rich resource for diabetes health and nutrition advice on everything from dietary guidelines, healthy recipes, results of the latest diabetes research studies, and other nutrition resources. Some of the information on the web is reliable and science-based, while at the same time misinformation abounds. How can you find the best nutrition information on the web?

- Determine the sponsor or owner of the web site you are browsing. Commercial interests should be clearly disclosed. This can clue you in to potential promotion of a certain medication or nutritional supplement.
- Look for nutrition web sites that post the credentials and affiliations of their content contributors and medical advisory board. Registered dietitians (RDs) and certified diabetes educators (CDEs) are highly qualified to provide Internet advice in the field of diabetes nutrition.
- Double-check information before you take it to heart. A reliable nutrition web site will back up its claims with

references to peer-reviewed medical literature and established scientific findings rather than testimonials.

- A good diabetes nutrition advice web site will note the date of the research it publishes and when the site was last updated. Credible web sites are updated often to communicate the most current scientific advice.
- Check for a seal of approval from a voluntary organization such as Health on the Net that requires adherence to quality guidelines.
- Log on to the following web sites to find high-quality diabetes nutrition information.
  - www.diabetes.org
  - www.niddk.nih.gov
  - www.nal.usda.gov/fnic
  - www.eatright.org
  - www.diabetes123.com
  - www.fbnr.com
  - www.healthtalk.com
  - www.mydiabetes.com

Ketones

Ketones are waste products that are made by your body when stored fat is used for energy. The body burns stored fat for energy when glucose is not available for use. People with diabetes can have ketones for several reasons. An inadequate amount of insulin can lead to an elevation in blood glucose. If there is not enough insulin, the body begins to break down body fat for energy. Physical or mental stress or illness such as the flu, a cold, or other infections may cause your body to get extra energy from fat. A low blood glucose caused by not enough food or too much insulin can lead to ketone production by the body. Also, inadequate insulin or food during exercise can cause your body to burn too much fat, resulting in ketones in your body. Likewise, ketones may occur with too few calories during pregnancy.

Ketones can build up in your blood, making it more acidic and causing an upset in your body's chemical balance. Ketones are passed into the urine so that the body can get rid of them. The body can also rid itself of one type of ketone, called acetone, through the lungs. This gives the breath a fruity odor.

Dangerously high levels of ketones can lead to ketoacidosis (sometimes called diabetic ketoacidosis or DKA), which is a warning sign that your diabetes is out of control or that you are getting sick. This life-threatening condition usually develops slowly with initial symptoms of thirst or a very dry mouth, frequent urination, high blood-glucose levels, and high levels of ketones in the urine. When vomiting occurs, ketoacidosis can develop in a few hours. If this condition worsens, you may have symptoms of extreme fatigue, dry or flushed skin, abdominal pain, nausea, vomiting, difficulty breathing, fruity odor on your breath, or confusion.

A simple urine test can detect ketones. Test for ketones during acute illness or stress, when your blood glucose levels are consistently over 240 mg/dl, when you have symptoms of ketoacidosis (nausea, vomiting, or stomach pain), and during pregnancy. When you are ill or when your blood glucose is more than 240 mg/dl, test for ketones every 4 to 6 hours. Avoid exercise when your urine tests show ketones and your blood glucose is high. Call your health care provider at once if your urine shows large ketones. Be sure and check with your health care provider about your individualized plan about when and how you should test for ketones.

Kidney Disease

The kidneys act as filters to clean the blood. They get rid of waste and extra fluid. In healthy kidneys, the filters let wastes pass out to your urine but keep useful nutrients in your blood. Diabetes can make your kidneys unhealthy, which can lead to kidney disease. Kidney disease is called nephropathy. High blood glucose and high blood pressure can damage the kidneys. When the kidneys are damaged, protein leaks out of the kidneys into the urine. Damaged kidneys do not do a good job of cleaning out waste and extra fluids. Not enough waste and fluids go out of the body as urine. Instead, they build up in your blood.

An early sign of kidney damage is when your kidneys leak small amounts of a protein called albumin into the urine. Eventually this leads to proteinuria, which means protein has leaked in the urine. Wastes products build up to toxic levels; this is called kidney failure or end-stage renal disease.

If you have advanced kidney disease, you may need dialysis, a treatment that takes waste products and extra fluid out of your body. There are two types of dialysis. You and your doctor will decide what type will work best for you. You may also be able to have a kidney transplant. This operation gives you a new kidney from a close family member, friend, or someone who matches your body.

You will know you have kidney problems only if your doctor tests your urine for protein. Do not wait for signs of kidney damage to have your urine tested. To prevent kidney disease, follow the tips below.

- Keep your blood glucose as close to normal as you can. Tight blood glucose control, more than anything else, can slow the progression of kidney disease.

- Control your blood pressure. High blood pressure makes the kidneys work harder, causing more damage. Ask your doctor what blood pressure numbers are best for you. Losing weight, eating less salt, and avoiding alcohol may also decrease your blood pressure. If you are on blood pressure medicine, take it faithfully.

- Follow the healthy eating plan you work out with your registered dietitian. You may be asked to limit your protein intake to slow down kidney disease. Foods high in protein include meat, fish, poultry, eggs, milk, cheese, legumes, whole grains, nuts, and seeds.

- Have your kidneys checked at least once a year by having your urine tested for small amounts of protein.

- See a doctor right away if you think you have a bladder or kidney infection.

If you develop kidney disease, you may be asked to follow a meal plan low in sodium, potassium, and protein. This is sometimes referred to as a renal diet. If you are on a renal diet, follow the general guidelines below.

- Eat the correct number of servings of protein foods. The body may use animal protein in a different way than the protein found in vegetables and grains.
- Watch the amount of potassium you eat. Potassium is a mineral found in salt substitutes, some fruits, vegetables, milk, chocolate, and nuts. Too much potassium can build up in your blood and be harmful to your heart. (Too little potassium is also harmful to your heart.)
- Limit how much you drink. Fluids build up quickly in your body when your kidneys aren't working.
- Avoid too much salt. Salty foods make you thirsty and cause your body to hold water.
- Limit foods high in phosphorus such as milk, cheese, nuts, dried beans, and soft drinks. Too much phosphorus in your blood causes calcium to be pulled from your bones. Calcium helps keep bones strong and healthy. To prevent bone problems, your doctor may give you special medicines.

Useful References

Web Site

www.nhlbi.nih.gov

Book

The Uncomplicated Guide to Diabetes Complications by Marvin E. Levin and Michael A. Pfeifer. Published by the American Diabetes Association, 1998.

Legumes

Legumes are a large family of plants distinguished by their seed-bearing pods and include common beans (such as navy, kidney, and pinto beans), common peas, soybeans, and peanuts. Because of their nutritional composition, legumes can play an important role in diabetes meal plans. All legumes are rich sources of plant protein, fiber, vitamins, and minerals. Common beans and peas are naturally low in fat. Because legumes are plant foods, they are cholesterol free. Legumes are naturally low in sodium, but canned beans may contain a significant amount of sodium, added during the canning process.

Research has shown that including 1 1/2 to 2 1/2 cups of cooked common beans in a diabetes meal plan can improve diabetes control. Beans have a low glycemic index, meaning they result in a minimal rise in blood glucose after they're eaten. The soluble fiber in beans can lower blood cholesterol and decrease the risk of heart disease, a major risk factor for people with diabetes. Beans can also delay hunger pangs after you eat them, making them helpful for weight control if you have type 2 diabetes.

Beans are recommended in all the major meal planning approaches for diabetes. One-half cup of beans and peas (garbanzo, pinto, kidney, white, split, and black-eyed) count as one starch exchange, plus one very lean meat exchange in *Exchange Lists for Meal Planning.* If you use *Carbohydrate Counting*, 1/2 cup of beans and peas equals one carbohydrate choice or 15 grams of carbohydrate. Because beans are rich in fiber, you may need to subtract their fiber content from the total grams of carbohydrate to determine how much carbohydrate is actually available to affect your blood glucose (see page 34).

Low-Carbohydrate Diets

Low-carbohydrate, high-protein diets, with their unlimited bacon, eggs, double cheeseburgers, and steak, have been popularly praised as weight loss wonders. People with diabetes should be extra cautious about jumping on the low-carbohydrate bandwagon, though. Low-carbohydrate diet promoters claim that carbohydrates in our diet are harmful because they increase insulin levels, which may lead to weight gain, elevated blood fats, high blood pressure, increased appetite, and mood changes, as well as diabetes. However, science proves that it isn't carbohydrate per se that causes these problems, but the calories from a variety of excess foods that make us put on the pounds and develop health risks.

Low-carbohydrate diets may cause weight loss because their strict meal plans are low in calories (1000 to 1400 calories daily) with a carbohydrate deficit that can lead to an unhealthy loss of muscle tissue and water. Low-carbohydrate diets also promote ketosis, the breakdown of body fat. People with diabetes should be aware that ketosis can become a serious medical situation. Both ketosis and the water loss from muscle tissue breakdown can also stress the kidneys. Low-carbohydrate, high-protein diets are often high in animal fat, which increases risk of heart disease. Other side effects from low-carbohydrate diets include constipation, dehydration, dizziness, fatigue, low blood pressure, nausea, "keto breath," and vitamin and mineral deficiencies.

Our bodies require carbohydrate for energy. Studies support the importance of including foods containing carbohydrate from whole grains, fruits, vegetables, and milk in the diet. Whether your diet should be low or high in carbohydrate is based on your individual health goals. The total amount of carbohydrate in meals or snacks, not the source or type of carbohydrate, is the first priority.

Meal Planning

Your meal plan is the cornerstone of your diabetes treatment, whether you have type 1, type 2, or gestational diabetes. Think of your meal plan as a series of lifestyle changes for long-term good health, rather than a short-term diet you go on and then off. Healthy eating is for life!

The key to a successful meal plan is individualization. A registered dietitian will work with you, learning more about your diabetes, treatment goals, and lifestyle to design the plan that works best for you. Rather than a preprinted "diet sheet," your meal plan should be tailored to your needs.

A good meal plan is based as closely as possible on your typical food intake, with a few changes made to improve blood glucose control. Your registered dietitian will help determine how many calories you need, the amount and spacing of your carbohydrate intake throughout the day, how many grams of fat you need, and how to adjust your food or medications when you exercise. Your meals and snacks should be coordinated with the action of your insulin or oral diabetes medication. The meal plan your dietitian designs is a template for whatever approach you'll be using, from carbohydrate counting to the food pyramid.

A perfectly designed meal plan won't do a bit of good if you can't put it into practice every day. You may want to budget time and money for a registered dietitian to design menus based on your meal plan and favorite foods. Other options include the American Diabetes Association *Month of Meals* books, a series that provides you with a set of menus for a month that can be mixed and matched to meet your individual nutrition needs. This approach may work well for you as a starting point, especially if you're the type of person who says "Just tell me what I can and can't eat."

Be aware that your meal plan should not be set in stone. In fact, it's a good idea to visit your registered dietitian regularly to update your meal plan, particularly if you've had a change in lifestyle or diabetes management goals.

Useful References

- **Books**

Month of Meals Cookbook Series: Classic Cooking, Ethnic Delights, Old-Time Favorites, Meals in Minutes, Vegetarian Pleasures. Published by the American Diabetes Association, 1998.

Medical Foods

An increased number of modified foods and nutritional products have been developed for the management of diabetes. Medical snack bars claiming to reduce hypoglycemia risk or decrease postprandial blood glucose are examples. Some bars are high in protein and low in carbohydrate. Others contain modified carbohydrate sources or soluble fiber. Some snack bars contain resistant starch, which is not digested and therefore not absorbed as glucose. Several of the bars are fortified with vitamins, minerals, and other nutrients and claim to be nutritionally complete. Liquid meal replacements are also marketed for people with diabetes.

Medical snack bars contain a range of carbohydrate, protein, and fat. Read Nutrition Facts on food labels to determine the nutrient content and how they will fit into your meal plan. The snack bars come in a variety of flavors and can be used as your evening snack to reduce the risk of nighttime and early morning hypoglycemia. Some companies advertise their snack bars to be used as a snack or meal replacement. Blood glucose monitoring will help you determine the effect these snack bars have on your blood glucose levels. Consider their cost, taste, and nutritional composition when you discuss using them with your diabetes care providers.

Medical Nutrition Therapy

Medical nutrition therapy (MNT) is a term that defines specific nutrition services to treat illness, injury, or a medical condition. It involves the whole spectrum of what was formerly known as diabetes nutrition education: assessment of your current nutritional status, setting nutrition goals, developing a nutrition treatment plan, and evaluating the results of the plan. Medical nutrition therapy is recognized as the cornerstone of treatment for diabetes, with medication, physical activity, and blood glucose monitoring also playing important roles. Medical nutrition therapy, implemented by a registered dietitian, provides you with several valuable benefits including reducing the amount of medication you need, decreasing the number of hospital admissions and the length of hospital stays, reducing painful and dangerous complications, and improving your quality of life.

The evidence supporting the significant role of medical nutrition therapy in the management of chronic disease is so strong that Congress passed legislation in 2000 to provide Medicare medical nutrition therapy coverage for individuals with diabetes or renal disease effective January 1, 2002. Health care plans and insurance carriers may also cover the cost of nutrition counseling, a real bargain for an individual with diabetes.

Metabolism

Metabolism is a process by which cells chemically change food so that it can be used to keep the body alive. Insulin from the pancreas is necessary for the metabolism of food. During normal fuel metabolism the body maintains:

- Blood glucose concentrations within normal ranges.
- An adequate supply of emergency carbohydrate in the form of glycogen in the liver and muscle.
- An adequate supply of protein for body functions and storage.

When food is eaten:

- The brain and other organs use some of the glucose that has been absorbed from the gastrointestinal tract.
- Unused glucose is stored in the liver, muscle, and fat tissues.
- Insulin levels are high to store glucose.

After food is absorbed:

- Insulin levels decrease.
- Energy storage from food ends.
- Carbohydrate and fat stored are mobilized to produce energy and maintain blood glucose levels.

Metabolism in people with diabetes involves:

- Reduced insulin activity due to lack of insulin (type 1 diabetes) or insulin resistance (type 2 diabetes).
- Disrupted connection between the amount of glucose entering (food eaten) and glucose leaving (used energy), resulting in hyperglycemia.

Achieving target blood glucose levels through insulin injections in people with type 1 diabetes and oral medications and/or insulin injections in people with type 2 diabetes restores normal fuel metabolism, in combination with meal planning and physical activity.

National Diabetes Education Program (NDEP)

The National Diabetes Education Program (NDEP) is a federally sponsored health initiative that encourages people with diabetes to control their blood glucose levels. The campaign raises awareness about the importance of controlling diabetes, especially among minority groups. The messages are targeted to people with diabetes, the general public, minority populations, health care providers, payers, and policy makers. The goal of the program is to improve the treatment and outcomes for people with diabetes, to promote early diagnosis, and, ultimately, to prevent the onset of diabetes.

Useful Reference

- **Web Site**
  http://ndep.nih.gov

"New Wave" Nutrition Definitions

Today's news is full of stories about cutting-edge approaches to nutrition, some of which you may be considering as part of your diabetes treatment plan. Here are a few definitions to guide you through the maze of "new wave" nutrition.

- **Alternative and Complementary Therapies.** These terms cover those treatments and healthcare practices not taught widely in medical schools, not generally used in hospitals, and not usually reimbursed by medical insurance companies. Some alternative and complementary therapies used to manage diabetes include acupuncture, used to relieve the chronic pain from neuropathy (diabetes nerve damage), and biofeedback or guided imagery, in which a person with diabetes thinks of images of controlling or curing their condition. Herbal, vitamin, and mineral supplements are also sometimes categorized as alternative or complementary therapies. A therapy is termed "alternative" if it is used alone for treatment or "complementary" if it is used in addition to conventional medical treatments.

- **Functional Foods.** Functional foods may provide health benefits beyond basic nutrition due to their active food components. These can be whole foods such as tomatoes, which contain lycopene, a compound that may prevent some forms of cancer. Functional foods can also include foods that have been fortified with nutrients or enhanced with phytochemicals. Probiotics, a form of functional foods, are live microbial food supplements that have a beneficial effect on intestinal microbial balance.

- **Organic Foods.** Organically produced foods have been treated with little or no chemicals or synthetic pesticides during the growing cycle. Some people believe organic foods are healthier and taste better, although scientists do not consider them to be higher in nutrients than their non-organic counterparts. Government standards are now in place to regulate the production of organic foods, including detailed instructions for crops and animal products.

- **Phytochemicals.** Phytochemicals are chemical compounds produced by plants to protect themselves from viruses, bacteria, and fungi. Although their exact role in promoting health is uncertain, they may be helpful in protecting against some cancers, heart disease, and other health conditions. Scientists have identified more than 600 different phytochemicals, a few of which appear below.
  - Carotenoids (found in carrot, broccoli, winter squash, sweet potato, apricot, papaya, cantaloupe, mango, and dark leafy greens)
  - Indoles, sulphoraphane, and isothiocyanates (found in cabbage, cauliflower, broccoli, Brussels sprouts, and greens)
  - Phytosterols and isoflavones (found in soybeans, tofu, and dried beans)
  - Vitamin C (found in citrus fruits, sweet peppers, and tomatoes)
  - Allylic sulfides (found in garlic, onions, leeks, ginger, and chives)
  - Lycopene (found in watermelon, tomatoes, and pink grapefruit)
  - Ellagiac acid (found in grapes, apples, mangoes, and papaya)

You may see phytochemicals advertised in the form of supplement pills, but there's no proof that these are effective. It's best to include a wide variety of fruits, vegetables, and legumes as whole foods in your meal plan.

Useful References

- **Web Site**
  www.cyberdiet.com
- **Book**
  The American Dietetic Association's Complete Food & Nutrition Guide by Roberta Duyff. Published by The American Dietetic Association, 1998.

Nutrition Recommendations for People with Diabetes

The American Diabetes Association sets nutrition guidelines for people with diabetes. The 2001 Nutrition Recommendations are based on the strongest available scientific evidence. These goals are established to help people with diabetes make changes in nutrition and exercise habits to improve their diabetes control. Specific goals include:

- Maintain as near-normal blood glucose levels as possible.
- Achieve optimal blood lipid levels.
- Maintain blood pressure levels that reduce the risk for vascular disease.
- Prevent or treat acute and long-term complications of diabetes.
- Improve health through food choices and increased physical activity.

These nutrition recommendations are similar to those for people without diabetes. Contact your RD to help you set individual nutrition goals in each area.

- **Carbohydrate.** This is the main source of energy for your body. They include sugars, such as sucrose, fructose, and lactose; and large molecules, such as starch. In the body, most carbohydrates break down into glucose. People with diabetes should include foods containing carbohydrate such as whole grains, fruits, vegetables, and milk in their diet. The amount of carbohydrate recommended is based on the individual's treatment goals and eating habits.

- **Fat.** Intake of saturated fat (including trans fatty acids) should be less than 10% of total calories. However, some individuals with an LDL of greater than 100 mg/dl may benefit by reducing saturated fat to 7% of total calories. Polyunsaturated fat intake should be less than 10% of total calories. Total fat intake should be individualized based on eating habits and treatment goals.

- **Cholesterol.** Dietary cholesterol intake should be less than 300 milligrams per day. However, if your LDL cholesterol is greater than 100 mg/dl, you may benefit by lowering your dietary cholesterol to less than 200 mg/day.

- **Fiber.** The recommendation for fiber intake is the same as for the general public. Daily consumption of 20–35 grams of dietary fiber, both soluble and insoluble, from a wide variety of food sources is recommended. Large amounts of dietary fiber (about 50 grams per day) may decrease blood glucose, insulin, and blood fats.

- **Protein.** Intake for people with diabetes without kidney disease should be the same as for the general public, 15–20% of total daily calories. Protein foods such as lean meats, low-fat dairy products, and low-fat plant protein foods should be selected to maintain a low-fat diet.

- **Sodium.** Less than 2400 milligrams per day is recommended.

- **Vitamins and minerals.** When vitamin and mineral intake from the diet is adequate, there may be no need for additional supplementation. Daily calcium supplementation of 1000–1500 milligrams, especially in the elderly, may be needed to prevent bone disease. Folate supplementation is recommended in women of child-bearing age to prevent birth defects.

- **Alcohol**. If individuals choose to drink, daily intake should be limited to no more than 1 drink for women and 2 drinks for men. One drink is 12 ounces of beer, 5 ounces of wine, or 1 1/2 ounces of spirits.

Useful References

- **Web Sites**
  www.diabetes.org
  www.eatright.org

Obesity

Aiming for a healthy weight is important to achieve good health and reduce the risk of many chronic diseases, including diabetes, high blood pressure, high blood cholesterol, heart disease, stroke, arthritis, breathing problems, and certain types of cancer. Reaching and maintaining a healthy weight can improve blood glucose tolerance and blood lipid levels, which are crucial for people with diabetes.

A healthy weight is not one number but a range that takes into consideration your age, gender, body shape, and location of body fat. For people with diabetes, the American Diabetes Association recommends a weight that is achievable and maintainable, both in the short and long term. This means that setting a realistic weight goal from the start and maintaining a healthy weight permanently is best for health, not an ongoing weight cycle of ups and downs.

There are several methods to evaluate our body weight.

- **Desirable Body Weight.** Follow these steps to determine desirable body weight for a medium-frame person. For women: start with 100 pounds for the first five feet of height. Add five pounds for each additional inch. For men: start with 106 pounds for the first five feet of height. Add six pounds for each additional inch. For small frames, subtract 10% and for large frames, add 10%.

- **Body Mass Index (BMI).** This method evaluates your weight in relation to your height. To find your BMI, multiply your weight in pounds by 705. Divide your answer by your height in inches. Divide this answer by your height again. A BMI from 18.5 up to 25 is considered healthy.
- **Waist-To-Hip Ratio.** Excess body fat that settles in the area around the waist puts a person at higher risk for health problems. To find your waist-to-hip ratio, measure your waist at its smallest point. Measure your hips at the largest part of your buttocks and hips. Divide your waist measurement by your hip measurement. For a healthy weight, the waist-to-hip ratio for most women should fall below 0.8; for men, below 0.95 is best.

Useful Reference

- **Web Site**
  www.usda.gov

Oral Diabetes Medicines

If you have type 2 diabetes, you may be amazed and overwhelmed by the astounding array of oral diabetes medicines available to help you control your blood glucose. Type 2 diabetes can be caused by a variety of problems with glucose metabolism: your pancreas doesn't produce enough insulin, your liver releases too much glucose, or your muscle cells don't readily take in glucose. Today, diabetes medications are being developed to target each problem area. You should be aware of the nutrition implications for each type of oral diabetes medication your physician prescribes.

The following oral diabetes medications have the potential to cause hypoglycemia, so work with your registered dietitian to plan for healthy snacks throughout the day and know the symptoms and treatment for low blood glucose (see page 146) if you are taking medicines from these classes.

- **Sulfonylureas.** Drugs in this class stimulate insulin secretion from the pancreas and include acetohexamide (Dymelor), chlorpropamide (Diabinese), glimepiride (Amaryl), glipizide (Glucotrol, Glucotrol XL), glyburide

(DiaBeta, Glynase PresTab, Micronase), tolazamide (Tolinase), and tolbutamide (Orinase).

- **Combination Sulfonylurea/Biguanide.** Glucovance is a combination of glyburide and metformin (see information below), so if you take this medication, you may need to plan for healthy snacks and know the symptoms and treatment for hypoglycemia.
- **Thiazolidinediones.** Rosiglitazone (Avandia) and pioglitazone (Actos) are the major drugs in this class. They are often used in combination with other diabetes medications and work by making your tissues more sensitive to insulin.
- **Meglitinides.** Repaglinide (Prandin) helps prevent blood glucose from rising after a meal by stimulating insulin secretion from your pancreas. It should be taken 30 minutes before meals or large snacks and it may be taken in combination with other diabetes medicines.
- **D-phenylalanine (amino acid) Derivative.** Nateglinide (Starlix) is the first diabetes medication to be released in this new classification of drugs. It acts by stimulating short-acting insulin secretion from your pancreas after a meal or large snack in a similar fashion to the meglitinides, but more rapidly. Nateglinide can be taken in combination with metformin.

The following oral diabetes medications very rarely cause hypoglycemia when taken alone, but may cause low blood glucose if you take them with another medication that does.

- **Alpha-Glucosidase Inhibitors.** Drugs in this class include acarbose (Precose) and miglitol (Glyset). These drugs should be taken with the first bite of each meal. They control your blood glucose after meals by slowing down the digestion of carbohydrates. Acarbose and miglitol don't cause hypoglycemia or weight gain, but may cause you to experience gastrointestinal side effects.

- **Biguanides.** Metformin (Glucophage, Glucophage XR) is a biguanide. It works by preventing your liver from producing too much glucose, while making your body more sensitive to insulin. When used alone, these medicines very rarely cause hypoglycemia, but they can cause a loss of appetite and gastrointestinal side effects. You may need to start with a low dose, take it with meals, and build up slowly.

Although none of these oral diabetes medicines is "oral insulin," progress is being made in the development of an oral medication that slows the digestion of insulin if taken by mouth long enough to allow it to be absorbed into the bloodstream to lower blood glucose. Pilot studies into oral insulin are being done in both type 1 and type 2 diabetes. As with any medication, side effects are possible. Long-term data on the safety of the newer medications may not be available.

Useful Reference

- **Book**

  101 Medication Tips for People with Diabetes by Betsy Carlisle, Lisa Kroon, and Mary Anne Koda-Kimble. Published by the American Diabetes Association, 1999.

Osteoporosis

Osteoporosis is a condition of gradually weakening, brittle bones caused by lowered bone mass. Thin, frail bones break easily and are the number one cause of bone fractures of the spine, hip, and wrist in people over 45. Low calcium intake is one risk factor for osteoporosis. Osteoporosis affects both women and men, but is more common among women. At menopause, a woman's estrogen level drops dramatically, removing estrogen's protective effect on bones. Other risk factors for osteoporosis are family history; being a fair-skinned, small-framed white or Asian woman; lack of weight-bearing exercise; smoking and alcohol use; and early menopause.

Your body constantly breaks down and rebuilds bone, so you need to eat calcium-rich foods throughout your life. The amount of calcium you consume in childhood and adolescence influences the strength of your bones when you reach adulthood. But it is never too late to get enough calcium. Lifelong adequate calcium intake helps maintain bone health by increasing as much as genetically possible the amount of bone formed in the teens and early adult life and by helping to slow the rate of bone loss that occurs later in life. Follow these steps to keep your bones healthy:

- Get enough calcium. Eat at least three servings of calcium-rich foods every day, no matter what your age. All adult needs at least 800 milligrams of calcium a day. Adults over age 50 need 1200 milligrams per day. Teenagers need 1300 milligrams per day. Pregnant and nursing mothers may need additional calcium. To protect against osteoporosis, up to 1500 milligrams of calcium daily may be advised.
- Exercise regularly and include weight-bearing activities.
- Eat enough calories to maintain a healthy weight.
- Make sure you get enough vitamin D from sunshine and vitamin-D fortified milk, fish, and eggs. Vitamin D helps your body absorb and use calcium.
- Avoid smoking.
- Eat a balanced diet.
- Ask your physician about estrogen replacement therapy. A low dose of estrogen, typically given with progestin, helps slow bone loss.

Dairy foods such as milk, yogurt, cheese, ice cream, and cottage cheese supply most of the calcium in our diets. Other foods, such as deep-green leafy vegetables and fish with edible bones, provide significant amounts. Though leafy-green vegetables and grain products supply some calcium, they may also contain oxalates and phytates that bind with calcium, partially blocking their absorption. Many processed foods, such as orange juice and breakfast cereal, may be fortified with calcium.

CALCIUM IN FOODS

Food	Calcium (milligrams)
Yogurt, low-fat plain (1 cup)	415
Milk (1 cup)	295
Calcium-fortified orange juice (3/4 cup)	225
Cheese (1 oz)	205
Salmon, canned with edible bones (3 oz)	205
Broccoli (1 cup cooked)	135
Ice cream (1/2 cup)	85
Cottage cheese (1/2 cup)	75

The Food and Drug Administration allows foods or supplements high in calcium to make a nutrition claim on the food label about the link between calcium and osteoporosis. Typical foods with this health claim are low-fat milk, yogurt, tofu, calcium-fortified citrus drinks, and some calcium supplements.

Food sources of calcium are preferred over supplements. However, as an extra safeguard your health care professionals may recommend a calcium supplement. If you take a calcium supplement, take the calcium as a supplement, not as a replacement for food sources of calcium. Read the label to determine the amount of calcium the supplement contains. If you take two or three tablets daily, space them throughout the day to improve their absorption. Drink plenty of fluids with calcium supplements to avoid constipation. If you take your calcium supplement with milk, the lactose and vitamin D in the milk can help enhance absorption of the calcium.

Percent Daily Values

The Percent Daily Values (%DV) on the Nutrition Facts Panel of food labels tells you whether the nutrients (such as fat, sodium, and fiber) in a serving of food contribute a lot or a little to your total daily diet. The %DV shows you the percent (or how much) of the recommended daily amount of a nutrient is in a serving of food. By using the %DV, you can tell if this amount is high or low. They help you see how a food fits into an overall daily diet.

The %DVs are based on recommendations for a 2,000-calorie diet. Larger food packages also have the daily values for 2500 calories. Depending on your age, gender, and activity level, you may need more or less than 2000 calories. Whether or not you eat more or less than 2000 calories each day, you can still use the %DV as a frame of reference.

The %DV for total fat, saturated fat, cholesterol, sodium, total carbohydrate, and dietary fiber are required to be listed on labels. No daily reference value has been established for sugar because no recommendations have been made for the total amount of sugars to be eaten. A %DV for protein is required to be listed if a claim is made for protein. Otherwise, unless the food is meant for use by infants and children under 4 years old, a %DV for protein is not required.

The %DV for two vitamins, A and C, and two minerals, calcium and iron, must be listed. If a nutrition claim is made about a vitamin or mineral other than those required to be listed, the %DV in the food must be on the label.

In general, try to limit your total daily intake of fat, saturated fat, sodium, and cholesterol to less than 100%DV. Try to get enough essential nutrients such as calcium, iron, and vitamins A and C as well as other components such as dietary fiber. Try to average 100% for each one of these nutrients each day.

Eating a food with 5%DV or less means the food is fairly low in this nutrient. Try to select most foods with 5%DV or less for fat, saturated fat, sodium, and cholesterol. Foods with 20%DV or more means the food is fairly high in the nutrient. Try to select foods with more than 20%DV for calcium, iron, and vitamins A and C.

Useful References

- **Web Site**

  http://vm.cfsan.fda.gov/label.html

- **Book**

  Reading Food Labels—A Handbook for People with Diabetes by the American Diabetes Association and The American Dietetic Association, 1994.

Point or Counting Systems

A point or counting system is one approach to diabetes meal planning that keeps track of your intake of calories, carbohydrate, or fat. A variety of meal planning methods based on point or counting systems are currently used.

- **Calorie Point System.** This system is based on the concept of counting calorie points, with one point equaling 75 calories. Each portion size of a food choice is identified as containing a certain number of calorie points. For example, one hard-boiled egg equals about 75 calories or one point. Individuals work with a dietitian to determine a target number of points to eat at each meal and each snack. For example, a 1500-calorie diet would contain 20 points, to be divided throughout the day based on the diabetes medication being used. This approach to meal planning can be very useful if you have type 2 diabetes and need to control your weight; however, it doesn't include any emphasis on the carbohydrate content of foods, which may lead to fluctuations in blood glucose.

- **Carbohydrate Choice Method.** The carbohydrate choice method can be used for carbohydrate counting (see page 34) if you don't want to count the actual grams of carbohydrate you eat. The basic concept is that 1 carbohydrate choice is equal to 15 grams of carbohydrate. With that information in mind, you and your dietitian determine the number of carbohydrate choices you need at each meal and snack, then monitor blood glucose testing results to make changes as necessary to keep your blood glucose within target range. While not as accurate as the carbohydrate gram counting approach, it is simpler and can help you become more consistent in your carbohydrate intake.

- **Fat Counting.** The fat counting approach is useful if you need to control your weight or if you are trying to lower elevated blood lipids. You and the registered dietitian will determine your daily fat allowance and the number of fat grams you can eat at each meal and snack. Reference books, the Exchange Lists, and food labels can provide information about the fat grams in foods. By itself, fat counting is not a suitable approach to diabetes management, since it doesn't include any emphasis on the carbohydrate content of foods.

- **Weight Watchers 1-2-3 Success Point System.** Although not developed specifically for individuals with diabetes, this approach may be helpful if you have type 2 diabetes and need to control your weight. Once your daily point range is determined based on your current weight, then you are allowed to eat any food or beverage you choose as long as you remain within your point range. Foods are assigned points based on their calorie, fat, and fiber content; however, carbohydrate information is not emphasized, which may make it more difficult for you to achieve good blood glucose control.

Useful References

- **Web Site**

  www.weightwatchers.com

- **Book**

  The Diabetes Carbohydrate and Fat Gram Guide by Lea Ann Holzmeister. Published by The American Diabetes Association, 2000.

Portion Control

An extra bite of mashed potatoes, an additional dollop of sour cream, or a handful of cashews may not sound like much, but if you aren't aware of food portion sizes, you may find yourself facing elevated blood glucose levels, weight gain, and poor diabetes control. In all diabetes nutrition plans—from carbohydrate counting to the food guide pyramid—portion size is a crucial factor. Know the portion sizes your meal plan suggests, then take a closer look at what you're actually eating. The following tips will help you become more "size-wise."

- Stock your kitchen with the tools of the trade: measuring spoons, measuring cups for both liquids and solids, and a food scale. Use these tools until you train your eyes to judge proper portion sizes. Measuring out a 3/4 cup serving of cereal, rather than randomly pouring a bowlful, can make a big difference in carbohydrate and calorie content.
- Learn to estimate portion sizes of familiar foods in your own home by observation. Pour a measured amount of milk into a favorite glass and note the level it comes to

on the glass. You can either mark the glass at that spot or remember where it levels off in relation to the design of the glass for future reference. The same technique will work for any food as you become aware of the way a measured amount looks on a familiar plate. You don't need to measure your food every time you eat; visualize! Double-check yourself occasionally to prevent slipping back into "portion distortion."

- Keeping a food diary will enable you to be more attentive to what you actually are eating. (See page 105 for more information about food diaries.)
- Size up your servings by comparing them to familiar items:
  - A small baked potato is the size of a computer mouse.
  - A closed fist is about the size of a 1-cup serving of pasta, rice, fruit, or vegetable.
  - Half a tennis ball is about the size of 1/2 cup of vegetables or fruit. A one-cup serving of broccoli is the size of a light bulb.
  - Three ounces of meat, poultry, or fish is about the size of one deck of playing cards, the palm of a woman's hand, or a computer mouse.
  - One ounce of cheese is about the size of your thumb or four dice.
  - Your thumb is about the size of one tablespoon of salad dressing or peanut butter. The tip of your thumb is about one teaspoon.

Pregnancy

A healthy pregnancy for women with diabetes begins even before you find out you're pregnant! If you have type 1 or type 2 diabetes, a complete physical, good nutrition (including a folic acid supplement), and excellent blood glucose control before you become pregnant will help minimize any health risks to you or your baby. Because all of the baby's major organs are formed during the first six to eight weeks of pregnancy, it is essential that your blood glucose be well controlled during this time to lower your baby's risk of birth defects. Needless to say, frequent blood glucose monitoring and a healthy pregnancy meal plan are essential for a successful pregnancy with diabetes. The best pregnancy outcomes seem to occur when the pregnancy lasts 39 to 41 weeks and the baby weighs between about 6 1/2 and 8 1/2 pounds.

Your health care team will work with you to set target blood glucose levels for you during pregnancy. Keeping blood glucose within the target ranges will minimize the risk of birth defects and miscarriage during the first trimester, as well as prevent the baby from growing too large during the remainder of the pregnancy. The American Diabetes Association suggests the following whole blood glucose goals during pregnancy (add 15% to convert the numbers to plasma glucose levels, depending on the glucose meter you use):

- Fasting: 60–90 mg/dl
- Premeal: 60–105 mg/dl
- 1 hour after meals: 100–120 mg/dl
- 2–6 hours after meals: 60–120 mg/dl

Your nutrition goal while pregnant is to provide everything your baby needs to grow while keeping your blood glucose level in control. Your registered dietitian and diabetes team will want to see you frequently to assess your progress and design a meal plan based on the following considerations.

- **Calories.** You will probably require about 100 extra calories per day during the first trimester and an additional 300 calories per day during the remainder of your pregnancy to ensure the ideal weight gain for you and birth weight for your baby.
- **Weight gain.** The amount of weight you should gain during your pregnancy is based on your weight before you became pregnant. If you were underweight, you should gain 28–40 pounds; if you were normal weight, you should gain 25–35 pounds; and if you were overweight, you should gain 15–25 pounds. How slowly or quickly you gain the weight is important too. You should gain slowly during the first trimester, then gain more weight during the second and third trimesters.
- **Vitamins and minerals.** Iron, zinc, and calcium are especially important during pregnancy. Ideally, if you eat a well-balanced diet with about 60 grams of protein a day, you don't require vita-

min and mineral supplementation. However, prenatal vitamins and minerals are often recommended as nutritional "insurance."

- **Meals and snacks.** Regularly-timed meals and snacks with a consistent intake of carbohydrate are important during pregnancy with diabetes to prevent hypoglycemia. A bedtime snack is especially important to prevent hypoglycemia during the night and urine ketones in the morning. Your meal plan should be adjusted frequently based on your blood glucose monitoring results, food habits and pregnancy progress.

- **Other nutritional considerations.**
  - At this time, research shows that the four most common **sugar substitutes** (acesulfame K, aspartame, saccharin, and sucralose) are safe to use during pregnancy, in moderation. Saccharin does cross the placenta and can reach the baby, but there is no evidence that it causes ill effects.
  - You should avoid drinking **alcohol** during pregnancy, because as in a pregnancy without diabetes, alcohol can cause birth defects.
  - Speak with your health care team about the amount of the stimulant **caffeine** you should consume.
  - Pregnant women should avoid **raw fish** to reduce the risk of viral and bacterial illness. In addition, new research suggests that pregnant women and nursing mothers should not eat shark, swordfish, king mackerel, and tilefish because the methyl mercury they contain may harm the unborn baby's developing nervous system.

Anyone with diabetes can benefit from an individualized meal plan designed with the help of a registered dietitian, but good nutrition is especially important for the health of a pregnant woman and her unborn baby. For more specific information about gestational diabetes (diabetes that occurs only during pregnancy), see page 115.

Useful Reference

- **Book**

  Diabetes and Pregnancy: What to Expect. Published by the American Diabetes Association, 2000.

Preventing Diabetes

The risk factors associated with type 1 diabetes and type 2 diabetes are different. Type 1 diabetes is more common in whites than in other ethnic groups. Other risk factors for type 1 diabetes have yet to be revealed. Type 2 diabetes is more common in Asian American, Hispanic American, African American and Native American ethnic groups. However, for both type 1 and type 2 diabetes, having a family history of diabetes puts you at a higher risk for developing the disease.

The strongest evidence points to these environmental risk factors as contributing to the development of type 2 diabetes.

- Obesity, especially central fat storage above the hips (apple-shaped body)
- High-calorie diet
- Physical inactivity
- Low intake of whole grains and dietary fiber
- High blood pressure and abnormal blood fat levels (high triglyceride level and a low HDL cholesterol level)

- Being over 45 years of age
- Women with a history of gestational diabetes or having had a baby weighing more than nine pounds
- Impaired fasting glucose or impaired glucose tolerance

Two important prevention studies are under way, one examining the prevention of type 1 and one the prevention of type 2 diabetes.

The Diabetes Prevention Trial—Type 1 (DPT—1) is a nationwide study to see if we can prevent or delay type 1 diabetes using insulin injections or insulin capsules. Preliminary results show no effect using insulin injections. Diabetes has a genetic link; close relatives of people with the disease have an increased chance of developing it. All family members, including children, are eligible for a free test in this study to determine their risk of getting diabetes.

The Diabetes Prevention Program (DPP) is designed to study the effectiveness of two types of lifestyle interventions and medication in preventing or delaying the development of type 2 diabetes. This study compares intensive lifestyle interventions to standard lifestyle interventions. Lifestyle interventions include healthy eating, reduced fat intake, and increased physical activity.

If you are at high risk for developing type 2 diabetes:

- Increase your physical fitness. Be active every day for 20 to 30 minutes.
- Manage your weight. If you are overweight, try losing five to ten pounds. Even losing this small amount of weight will lower your risk for developing diabetes.
- Reduce your intake of total and saturated fat. Decreasing your fat intake will help you lose weight by decreasing your calorie intake. Decreasing your saturated fat intake can help improve your blood lipid levels.

- Increase your intake of whole grains and fiber. Whole-grain consumption may improve insulin resistance. A high-fiber diet rich in fruits and vegetables will help with weight management.
- Balance your lifestyle. Make time for healthy eating and physical activity. This could help prevent diabetes and prolong your life!

Useful References

Web Site

www.niddk.nih.gov

Book

What You Can Do To Prevent Diabetes: Simple Changes to Improve Your Life by Annette Maggi and Jackie Boucher. Published by John Wiley & Sons, Inc., 2000.

Protein

Protein, along with fat and carbohydrate, is one of the main nutrients in our foods. It is made up of different chemicals called amino acids and is important in repairing body cells and regulating a variety of body processes. The body uses protein for energy if not enough fat or carbohydrate is available. Meat, poultry, fish, eggs, milk, cheese, yogurt, soy, legumes, seeds, and nuts are the major sources of protein in our diet. Most adults in the United States eat much more protein than the amount the body needs, which is about 10–20% of the day's calories.

Because people with diabetes are at risk for kidney disease, protein intake is often a special concern. Eating extra protein may make the kidneys work harder to eliminate the protein waste products. This is one of the problems associated with a high-protein, low-carbohydrate diet. However, there is no evidence that extra protein causes kidney disease. You may want to consider eating less protein or changing from animal sources to plant sources of protein if you develop kidney disease. Choose lean meats, low-fat dairy products, and plant foods as your main protein sources.

Research is providing us with new information about the effects of protein in nutrition for diabetes. For example, contrary to prior belief, protein does not have half the effect on blood glucose as carbohydrate does. Therefore you needn't consider the protein content of your meal when calculating your premeal insulin dose. Protein was also once thought to slow the absorption of carbohydrates, leading to the advice to eat a protein food with a high carbohydrate snack such as fruit to keep blood glucose stable. This now appears to be untrue. Scientists have also found that protein does not raise blood glucose 3 to 4 hours later than carbohydrate does, so a high protein snack will not necessarily prevent hypoglycemia. A registered dietitian can keep you up to date on the latest research on protein and work with you to develop an individualized meal plan that contains all of the essential amino acids you need for good health.

Recipes

It may seem contradictory, but diet and weight loss books and cookbooks share the bestseller honors in most bookstores. Actually, it isn't all that surprising since any meal planning approach requires a steady supply of tasty, convenient, and healthy recipes for success. A quick Internet search reveals more than 1400 diabetes books, many of which are cookbooks. With so many cookbooks competing for your attention, you need a few tips to make smart selections.

- The American Diabetes Association sells a wide variety of cookbooks through its catalog, by phone at 1-800-232-6733, or at the first web site listed below. ADA cookbooks focus on everything from quick and easy meal preparation to making specialty foods such as soul food or great dinners for entertaining.
- The American Dietetic Association maintains a "Good Nutrition Reading List" with a special section for people with diabetes and their families. Check out their web site at www.eatright.org for cookbooks that have passed the tests of good nutrition and good taste.

- When you are skimming through a cookbook you are considering for purchase, look for helpful information such as portion size and nutrient analysis of the recipes. If you always find yourself rushing when it's time to prepare supper, choose cookbooks that feature simple lists of ingredients and minimal preparation time, or you'll acquire an entire shelf of cookbooks with recipes that sound great but don't fit your busy lifestyle.

You can modify favorite family recipes to fit your special meal planning needs by analyzing the ingredient list and looking for ways to eliminate or reduce their fat, sugar, or sodium content. Substitute modified foods such as low-sodium broth or water-packed fruit whenever you can. Change food preparation methods with tricks such as skimming the fat off stews and soups, baking foods rather than deep-frying them, or skipping the salt in the cooking water. Still too many calories or carbs per serving? Reduce the portion sizes until they meet the nutrient amount that is right for you. Your registered dietitian can provide you with more information on modifying recipes and calculating their food values so they can fit your individualized meal plan.

Useful References

■ **Web Sites**

http://store.diabetes.org
www.cyberdiet.com
www.niddk.nih.gov

Registered Dietitian

Meal planning is often considered the most challenging aspect of diabetes care. A registered dietitian (RD) is the nutrition expert on your diabetes team who can help you understand the role that food plays in your blood glucose control and offer you ideas and resources to manage your meal plan. Your physician may refer you to a registered dietitian for counseling, or you may find an RD at a local hospital, clinic, or health department; you may find one in private practice or through your county extension office. Like most professionals, RDs charge a fee based on their experience and other factors. Your health care plan or insurance carrier may cover the cost of nutrition counseling, because the weight loss and improved blood glucose control that result have been proven to reduce or eliminate expensive diabetes medicine and avoid future complications and health problems.

Ideally, the RD will spend anywhere from half an hour to two hours with you initially, learning about your lifestyle, medical history, and diabetes goals. The RD will then develop a meal plan based as closely as possible on your eating habits and food preferences. Together, you'll set diabetes goals in the areas of target blood glucose levels, optimal blood lipid levels, attaining a reasonable weight, and improving overall health through good nutrition. Follow-up visits can be scheduled to answer questions and further refine your goals. Children with diabetes can benefit from a follow-up visit every three to six months; adults should ideally see the RD every six to 12 months to assess their progress.

Anyone can call themselves a "nutritionist," but for the most reliable nutrition information you should seek a credentialed registered dietitian, who has been registered by the Commission on Dietetic Registration of The American Dietetic Association (see page 7). An RD must earn a bachelor's degree in nutrition or a related field from an accredited college or university, complete an ADA-approved post-graduate training program, and pass an extensive registration exam. After registration, RDs are required to stay current with continuing education. In addition, many states now also require RDs to be licensed by their state. While all RDs should have a good understanding of the basic nutrition recommendations for diabetes, you may want to consult with an RD who specializes in diabetes management and is a Certified Diabetes Educator (CDE), certified by the National Certification Board for Diabetes Educators (see page 43).

Resistant Starch

Resistant starch is a category of food carbohydrate that is not completely digested by the body and therefore doesn't raise blood glucose in the same way as other carbohydrate foods do. After you eat resistant starch, blood glucose and insulin levels don't rise as much when compared to more digestible starches. Examples of whole foods containing resistant starch are legumes (such as lentils and soybeans) and cornstarch. Cornstarch may be modified to enhance its resistant starch content. While resistant starch has been incorporated into bedtime snack bar products aimed at reducing the incidence of nighttime hypoglycemia, there is currently no indication of long-term benefit.

Restaurant Dining

How often did you dine away from home last week? If you're anything like the average American, you found yourself eating out at least four times. As restaurant dining becomes more of a routine and less of a special occasion, it's important for you to know how to make healthy food choices for your diabetes. Whether you're sitting down at a steak house, calling for a pizza delivery, or bringing home a sub sandwich, keep a few guidelines in mind.

- Don't eat out impulsively. Plan ahead and choose a restaurant that offers a variety of foods, including healthier choices. Become familiar with the menus at the restaurants you frequent most often. You'll be able to decide what to order before you arrive, knowing exactly how your favorite food items fit into your meal plan.
- Read the menu carefully, looking for foods that are grilled, baked, broiled, poached, steamed, stir-fried, or roasted. Foods prepared with these techniques are often lower in fat and calories.

- Don't be afraid to make special requests. Ask for salad dressing on the side, a baked potato instead of fries, or a small green salad instead of the usual high-fat sides of coleslaw or potato salad.
- Prepare to share. Restaurants are notorious for serving enormous portion sizes. Why not order an appetizer and salad, while your dining companion orders an entrée? Mix and match for a complete meal. Feel free to ask for a "to go" bag so you can enjoy leftovers at home.
- Try to balance your restaurant meal with your food for the rest of the day. If you didn't have a fruit or vegetable at lunch, add one to supper. A high-fat meal at noon means you should keep things lean in the evening.
- Timing is everything. If you are scheduled to take an insulin injection with your meal, you may want to take it after you get to the restaurant in case your meal is delayed. Expect the unexpected, such as a mix-up in your order or a long wait for your table. Carry a source of carbohydrate with you—glucose tablets, crackers, or dried fruit—to munch on while you wait or to treat hypoglycemia.
- See page 54 for more tips on convenience food if you're living life in the fast food lane.

Useful Reference

- **Book**

  The American Diabetes Association Guide to Healthy Restaurant Eating by Hope Warshaw. Published by the American Diabetes Association, 1998.

Sick Days

Whether you're suffering from the flu, a virus, or a foodborne illness, being prepared is the key to coping with your diabetes and blood sugar control. Talk to your diabetes care team to learn the specific sick day guidelines you should follow. You may be asked to check your blood glucose levels at least every four hours and check your urine for ketones if your blood sugar levels are higher than 240 mg/dl or if you experience gastrointestinal symptoms. Ketones in the urine mean the body is breaking down fat stores for energy, which can lead to serious consequences if not properly treated.

You may not feel like eating or drinking, but it is important to sip liquids to help prevent dehydration. Try to take at least 1/2 cup of a calorie-free, caffeine-free liquid every 1/2 hour. If you can't eat solid foods, stick to your meal plan as closely as possible by substituting soft foods or beverages that contain carbohydrate. Suggested foods and amounts to replace one serving (15 grams) of carbohydrate include:

- 1/3 to 1/2 cup fruit juice
- 1/2 cup regular (not sugar-free) soft drink

- 1/2 cup regular gelatin
- 1/2 cup cooked cereal
- 1/2 cup vanilla ice cream
- 1 cup broth-based soup

Even if you are not eating and drinking normally, you will need to continue to take your insulin or diabetes medications unless instructed differently by your physician. Know when you should call your physician for advice. Most physicians recommend that you call them if you cannot keep down food, liquids, or diabetes medications; if your illness lasts more than 24 hours; if your temperature is over 101°F; if your blood glucose levels (at least two consecutive checks) remain outside the goals set previously for sick day management; or if your urine ketone test shows moderate to large ketones.

Snacks

In the past, everyone with diabetes was instructed to eat a diet composed of three meals and three snacks, regardless of their personal eating habits, diabetes medications, or health care goals. Now, individualization is the key to successful snack attacks that provide energy and prevent low blood glucose.

- People with diabetes who are taking one or two insulin shots with an intermediate acting insulin (NPH or Lente) may require between-meal snacks to provide the body with fuel and prevent low blood glucose reactions. If you're on an insulin pump or taking multiple daily insulin injections of a rapid-acting insulin, you may not require snacks at all because you'll take your insulin only at the time you actually eat.

- If you have type 2 diabetes and are diet-controlled or are taking oral diabetes medications, you may not want to snack between meals to promote weight loss and improve blood glucose levels. (See page 183 for more information about oral diabetes medications.)

Snacks can make a good eating plan even better. Choose snacks from the same healthy foods you eat at meals, concentrating on how the total amount of carbohydrate in the snack fits into your meal plan. You may want to try a piece of fruit, graham crackers, air-popped popcorn, low-fat yogurt mixed with whole grain cereal, or pretzels dipped in low-fat dip. To make a snack more substantial, add a source of protein such as low-fat milk, peanut butter, or low-fat cheese. You may want to carry a snack with you in case of delayed meals or unexpected schedule changes so you won't experience hypoglycemia or be tempted to grab the closest food, whether it's healthy or not.

Work with your registered dietitian to determine the best snacks for you, based on your blood glucose levels, eating habits, and diabetes goals.

Useful Reference

- **Book**
  The Diabetes Snack, Munch, Nibble, and Nosh Book by Ruth Glick. Published by the American Diabetes Association, 1998.

Sodium

Although the terms salt and sodium are commonly interchanged for one another, they aren't the same things. Table salt is actually the common name for sodium chloride, which is 40% sodium and 60% chloride. We require a certain amount of sodium in our diet, but excess sodium intake is linked to hypertension (high blood pressure), particularly in people with type 2 diabetes who may be more sodium sensitive than the general population.

It's difficult to assess your individual sodium sensitivity, so the nutrition recommendations for sodium for people with diabetes are the same as for the general population: less than 2400 mg sodium per day.

Where does the sodium in your diet come from? One teaspoon of table salt contains about 2400 mg of sodium, but the vast majority of sodium in our diet comes from processed foods such as canned foods, convenience foods, and salty snack foods. A preference for salty foods is acquired, but you can lower your sodium intake by trying the following tips.

- Read the Nutrition Facts panel on all the foods you buy to determine the amount of sodium in one serving of a food. If you are following a sodium-restricted diet, you may want to eat only foods with less than 400 mg sodium per single serving of food or less than 800 mg sodium per entrée or convenience meal.
- Choose fresh meats, fruits, and vegetables rather than high-sodium processed, canned, and convenience foods.
- Prepare your foods with less salt and season with a variety of herbs and spices. Read the food label carefully if you decide to use an herb/spice blend; some of these products may contain a significant amount of sodium.
- Go easy on the high-sodium condiments such as pickles, mustard, ketchup, soy sauce, and tartar sauce.

A word about salt substitutes: they may not be for you, particularly if you have kidney problems. Many salt substitutes contain the mineral potassium in place of sodium, which may be harmful if your kidneys aren't able to eliminate excess levels of potassium. Some salt substitutes don't give the same flavor as salt and may taste sharp or bitter. If you can shift gradually to a lower sodium intake, your desire for salty tastes will also be reduced.

Soy

An abundance of soy products are showing up in your supermarket. Are you familiar with soy's health benefits and how to put them to work in your kitchen? Soy products are derived from the soybean, which in itself is a nutrition powerhouse. Soybeans are a rich source of plant protein, fiber, vitamins, and minerals. The fat in soybeans is polyunsaturated, which is a bonus for heart health.

Soy protein may help prevent several diseases. Scientists think that the health benefits in soy products come from isoflavones, although research is still needed to determine exactly how these plant hormones work. Soy protein helps lower blood cholesterol, reducing the risk for heart disease. It may also play a role in preventing some forms of cancer, reducing the symptoms of menopause, and preventing osteoporosis. Substituting soy protein for animal protein in the diets of individuals with diabetes has been proposed as a way to lower the risk of diabetic nephropathy (kidney disease).

Most soy products are very mild in flavor and actually take on the taste of whatever you prepare them with. Here's the scoop on the most commonly available soy products.

- **Soy Milk.** Soy milk is a non-dairy beverage made from crushed soybeans. Although it's a good source of protein, be sure to choose a brand that is fortified with calcium, vitamin A, and vitamin D. One cup of soy milk is equal to a medium-fat meat exchange in the *Exchange Lists for Meal Planning.*
- **Tempeh.** Tempeh is a cake-form of soy made from fermented soybeans mixed with a grain source. It is a bit more flavorful than tofu and can be broiled, grilled, stir-fried, and used in casseroles. On the *Exchange Lists for Meal Planning,* 1/4 cup of tempeh is equal to a medium-fat meat exchange.
- **Textured Soy Protein.** Textured soy protein is a granular form of soy flour that can be added to main dishes as a protein boost or meat extender. Check the food label for nutrition information.
- **Tofu.** Tofu is the most familiar form of soy. It is a cheese-like curd made from soy milk and pressed into a cake shape. Different types of tofu are available to be used in different ways: "soft" or "silken" for blending into shakes and sauces, "medium" for mashing into pudding or cheesecake, and "firm," which can be sliced and grilled, marinated and stir-fried, or crumbled into a vegetarian chili or lasagna. Tofu is an excellent source of protein, but with about one-half of its calories coming from fat, you may be interested in a reduced-fat version. Four ounces or 1/2 cup of tofu is listed as one medium-fat meat exchange on the *Exchange Lists for Meal Planning.*

A variety of products from burgers to hot dogs made with soy is also available. Check the food label to be sure that processing hasn't made them too high in fat or sodium.

Special Occasions

The special occasions in your life range from birthdays to holidays to vacations. These are times to celebrate—and often times that make it difficult to follow your diabetes meal plan. While your diabetes management on an everyday basis is what matters the most in the long run, the following tips will help you survive special occasions while keeping your diabetes in control.

- Focus on the reason for the special occasion you are celebrating. Whether it's a promotion at work or a new baby, food should be only one small part of the celebration. Rather than making meals the centerpiece of the event, focus on enjoying family and friends.
- Don't let a special occasion become an excuse to ease up on your physical activity routine. Although you may feel too busy to exercise during the holidays, physical activity is a great way to reduce stress and improve blood glucose control. You may have to be more creative to include the physical activity you need. Try a family walk after eating Christmas dinner or playing Frisbee on the beach during vacation to get you moving and burn extra calories!

- A party won't be a diabetes diet disaster if you follow a few simple strategies. Don't ever go to a party hungry. If you eat a small snack before you go, you won't be tempted to devour the first thing you see on the buffet table. Take a moment to look over the buffet table carefully before making your choices. Don't waste calories and carbohydrate grams on foods you don't really enjoy. Finally, socialize away from the food table rather than standing next to it. Unconscious nibbling adds up.

- Favorite holiday recipes can be modified to make them healthier and still take a place of honor on your table without sacrificing taste. Use lighter cooking methods or substitute low-fat ingredients in dips and desserts. Rethink your traditional holiday menu. Why not serve baked squash rather than the tried and true candied sweet potatoes?

- If you plan to drink alcohol on a special occasion, do so knowing that it may affect your blood glucose. See page 3 for more information about alcohol.

- Be realistic about your diabetes control when you are enjoying a special occasion. Instead of trying to lose weight over the holidays or on vacation, focus on the goal of maintaining your weight and keeping your blood glucose in good control.

Sugar Alcohols

Sugar alcohols, also called polyols, are ingredients used in foods as sweeteners and/or bulking agents. Besides adding sweetness, sugar alcohols also add texture, help food stay moist, prevent browning when food is heated, and give a cooling effect to the taste of food. The term alcohol refers to their chemical structure. They do not contain ethanol as alcoholic beverages do.

Hydrogenated starch (HSH), isomalt, lactitol, maltitol, mannitol, sorbitol, xylitol, and erythritol are examples of sugar alcohols. Because sugar alcohols are only partially absorbed from the small intestine, they contain 1–3 calories per gram compared to 4 calories per gram in other sugars.

Sugar alcohols are used to sweeten a variety of foods, such as candy, chewing gum, baked goods, ice cream, and fruit spreads. They are also found in toothpaste, mouthwash, and medications, including cough syrups and throat lozenges. They are often used in the candies and cookies found in the "dietetic" section of the supermarket. These foods are not calorie- or carbohydrate-free. The calorie and carbohydrate savings when sugar alcohols are used instead of other sugar are not likely to produce a lower glucose response than other sugars. Therefore, there is little advantage to using these agents instead of other calorie-containing sweeteners.

While sugar alcohols have been determined by the FDA as safe for use as food additives, the use of certain polyols in foods triggers the need for a food "warning" concerning excess consumption and the laxative effect they have. Because sugar alcohols are not completely digested in the stomach, you may experience uncomfortable side effects such as diarrhea, intestinal cramping, or gas if you eat too much of them. Read ingredient lists on food labels to identify the sweetening agents used. Test your blood glucose to evaluate their effect on your diabetes control.

Useful Reference

- **Book**
  A Guide to Fitting Foods with Sugar Substitutes and Fat Replacers Into Your Meal Plan by the American Diabetes Association, 1998.

Sugar Substitutes

Nonnutritive sugar substitutes provide the sweet taste of sugar with far fewer calories and carbohydrate. Therefore, they don't raise blood glucose levels. Currently, four nonnutritive sweeteners have been approved by the United States Food and Drug Administration for use in the United States.

- Acesulfame K (*Sweet One, Sunette*): 200 times sweeter than table sugar. Suitable for cooking and baking.
- Aspartame (*NutraSweet, Equal*): 180–220 times sweeter than table sugar. May change flavor when heated. Aspartame breaks down into the amino acid phenylalanine, which should be noted by individuals with phenylketonuria (PKU).
- Saccharin (*Sweet'N Low*): 300 times sweeter than table sugar. Suitable for cooking and baking. Previously there were concerns regarding saccharin and bladder cancer, but it has been dropped from the list of known or likely carcinogens.

- Sucralose (*Splenda*): 600 times sweeter than table sugar. Made from sugar that has been changed so it's not absorbed by the body. Suitable for cooking and baking.

These products have undergone extensive safety testing and Acceptable Daily Intake (ADI) levels have been set for most of them. The ADI levels, which are far more than anyone would typically eat, specify the amount that can be eaten in a lifetime without any effect on health. Research has shown that all four sugar substitutes are safe for use during pregnancy; however, moderation is advised. Saccharin can cross the placenta, but there is no evidence that it causes ill effects.

Sugar substitutes are sold in both packets and in bulk for cooking at home. Some sugar substitutes work better in cold beverages than in cooking or baked goods. Read the product information and use recipes provided by the manufacturer for the best results.

Sugar substitutes are used in everything from diet sodas to desserts. Foods made with sugar substitutes are not necessarily calorie-free or carbohydrate-free. Check the food information label to see which sugar substitutes are used in a particular product and the total carbohydrate content per serving of the product. You may find that some foods and beverages are sweetened with a blend of sugar substitutes and sugar, so their calorie and carbohydrate content must also be included in your allowance for the day.

Sugar alcohols and fructose are known as nutritive sweeteners, another form of sugar substitute that contains calories and may raise your blood glucose. (See page 222 and page 226 for more information.)

Sugars and Sweets

For many years, the standard dietary advice for people with diabetes was to avoid eating sugar. This was based on the belief that eating sugar would cause blood glucose levels to rise much more rapidly than eating other types of carbohydrates, such as bread or potatoes. Research has since shown that all carbohydrates, whether from sugars or starches, will raise blood glucose levels in a similar way. Your blood glucose level is influenced mainly by the total amount of carbohydrate you eat, rather than the source of the carbohydrate. This means that you can include some sugars and sweets in your meal plan and stay in control of your blood glucose, as long as you account for the calorie and carbohydrate content.

Sugars are found naturally in some foods such as fruit (fructose) and milk (lactose). Our bodies cannot distinguish between natural sugars and sugars such as table sugar (sucrose) that have been added to food. Other examples of sugars include honey, dextrin, malt, molasses, syrup (such as corn syrup, high-fructose corn syrup, and maple syrup), corn sweeteners, brown sugar, powdered sugar, raw sugar, turbinado sugar, cane sugar, invert sugar, evaporated cane juice, and fruit juice concentrate. Check the food label information of a product to determine what types of sugar it contains, how much of the total carbohydrate is sugar, and the amount of total carbohydrate per serving. Be especially alert for words ending in "-ose" such as dextrose, glucose, and maltose.

All carbohydrates are made of chemical units. Sugars with one unit are called monosaccharides. Sugars with two units are called disaccharides. All sugars in foods contain four calories per gram and raise your blood glucose about the same way.

You may have noticed that many "diabetic" cookies and candies are sweetened with fructose, which is known as a nutritive sweetener because it contains calories and carbohydrate. Fructose has been found to cause a smaller rise in blood glucose levels than does glucose or sucrose, although eating large amounts of fructose may have negative effects on your blood lipids. Therefore, there is no advantage to using fructose in place of other sugars.

How much sugar can you include in your meal plan? There is no magic number of grams of sugar for the day, but people with diabetes should follow the same healthy eating guidelines as those without diabetes: choose beverages and foods to moderate your intake of sugar. Focus on the total carbohydrate intake for the day, rather than grams of sugar. If you want a sweet treat occasionally, substitute it for part of the carbohydrate in your meal plan instead of eating it in addition to your carbohydrate allowance. Remember that sugar and sweets have calories, but few vitamins or minerals. Foods made with lots of sugar are often high in fat and calories, which can affect your weight and blood lipids as well as your blood glucose. Eat small amounts of high sugar foods. If you decide to try a sweet treat, measure your blood glucose before and 1–2 hours after eating to note the effect a sugary food has on your blood glucose. Use that information to make smart sugar selections in the future.

Toddlers

Toddlers are trying to establish a sense of autonomy while exploring their surroundings. They do not have the cognitive skills to understand the need for structured eating habits and schedules and are reluctant to tolerate painful injections and blood tests. Parents of toddlers with diabetes take total responsibility for learning and managing the diabetes. The goal for diabetes care for infants and toddlers is to avoid very high and very low blood glucose levels. Symptoms of hypoglycemia in toddlers include crying, pallor, sweating, crankiness, and trembling. These symptoms are the best signal to test your child's blood glucose levels.

Growth slows down after the first year and toddlers may experience swings in their appetite. Consistent patterns of food intake are uncommon in toddlers, making blood glucose control difficult. Toddlers usually prefer to graze, eating small, frequent meals throughout the day. Toddlers are learning to feed themselves and selective eating is common. Avoid food hassles by offering age-appropriate portion sizes at meals and snacks.

Due to your child's large fluctuations in appetite and food selections, you may want to use rapid-acting insulin after the meal. Parents can learn carbohydrate counting and an insulin-to-carbohydrate ratio that meets their child's needs. Parents estimate food and carbohydrate intake and provide appropriate insulin dosing. Post-meal insulin dosing allows the insulin dose to change with the child's appetite, from meal to meal, and day to day without compromising blood glucose control. Frequent blood glucose monitoring is essential to identify blood glucose trends and prevent hypoglycemia.

Useful References

- **Web Sites**

  www.childrenwithdiabetes.com
  www.jdfcure.org

- **Books**

  Getting a Grip on Diabetes: Quick Tips & Techniques for Kids and Teens by Spike and Bo Nasmyth Loy. Published by the American Diabetes Association, 2001.

  Guide to Raising a Child with Diabetes, 2nd Edition by Linda Siminerio and Jean Betschart. Published by the American Diabetes Association, 2000.

  Sweet Kids: How to Balance Diabetes Control & Good Nutrition with Family Peace by Betty Brackenridge and Richard Rubin. Published by the American Diabetes Association, 1996.

Total Available Glucose

The protein, fat, and carbohydrate in our foods are eventually converted to glucose to be used by the body. Total available glucose (TAG) is a very precise meal planning approach that attempts to predict the way a certain food will affect your blood glucose based on its protein, fat, and carbohydrate content. Using this approach, foods are assigned a TAG value calculated by assuming that 100% of the carbohydrate content, 58% of the protein content, and 10% of the fat content of foods become glucose. However, recent research indicates that protein does not have the effect on blood glucose levels that was previously assumed, which may affect the way the TAG meal planning approach is used.

A typical 2200-calorie meal plan translates into about 325 TAG for the day. Foods are assigned TAG values; for example, one cup of whole milk has 16 TAG. In addition to calculating TAG, a glucose-to-insulin (G/I) ratio can be calculated to determine the amount of insulin required for metabolism of a particular food.

Although this meal planning approach is very precise, it is quite time-consuming and probably does not offer any advantages over carbohydrate counting (see page 34). If you would like to try the TAG meal planning approach, be prepared to schedule several sessions with a registered dietitian to learn and confidently apply it.

Travel

Whether you are traveling for the weekend or overseas for a month, it's important to take the time to plan ahead and be prepared. This is especially true for people with diabetes. Talk with travel agents, friends with diabetes who travel, and health care providers. Find out about the climate, culture, and food at your destination by checking local libraries and Internet sites. Contact the American Diabetes Association for a listing of recognized diabetes education programs and health care providers in the areas you will be traveling. Ask your health care provider to write prescriptions for your diabetes medicines so you will have extra to take with you and the ability to obtain more on the road.

If you are traveling to a different time zone, you will need to make adjustments in the time you take your medication and eat your meals. It is best to get accustomed to the new time zone you are visiting as quickly as possible. In some states or countries it customary to eat the evening meals late or have a large meal mid-day. You can make adjustments for this. Before you travel, check with your health care professionals for medication changes for different time zones and meal plan adjustments for varying meal times.

Eating on the road can be a real challenge to diabetes control and nutrition balance. Be ready for the unexpected, including cancelled flights, lost luggage, and illness. Pack supplies to treat low blood glucose and plenty of healthy snack foods. Bring portable snacks such as crackers, jar of peanut butter, canned single-serving fruit cups, tuna salad in a can, single serving dry cereal, granola bars, fresh fruit, popcorn cakes, and dried fruit. Keep snacks in resealable plastic bags to keep them fresh. Always have snacks and glucose products with you to treat low blood glucose.

Think ahead about your plans for physical activity during your trip. Compare this level of activity to your usual amount at home. Talk with your health care professionals about making adjustments in your meal plan and/or medications to keep your blood glucose levels in your target ranges.

Talk with your registered dietitian about how local dishes or native foods fit into your meal plan. Check on the availability of restaurants, markets, or other places to eat. Depending on your destination, you may eat all your meals out. Follow tips for healthy restaurant eating (see page 210). Restaurants usually serve large portions, which, if eaten, can add up to extra pounds quickly.

Depending on your mode of travel, keep the following tips in mind.

- **Travel by auto**. You are in control of your own schedule for meals and snacks. Keep a cooler in your car and store meals and snack items. Travel by car leaves you sitting for long periods. This can cause your blood glucose levels to increase. Stop frequently for stretch periods or short walks.

- **Travel by plane**. Be prepared for delayed or cancelled flights by carrying all your diabetes supplies and extra snacks with you at all times. Find out if and how much food will be served on your flight. Contact your airlines or travel agent in advance for special meal requests. Diabetic meals offered by airlines may not meet your meal plan needs. Carry water with you to keep you hydrated and avoid drinking excess alcohol and caffeine.

- **Travel by boat.** Most cruise lines offer flexible meal times and buffet-style eating. Request specific eating times and special meals if needed. Buffet-style eating encourages overeating. Have a plan for eating when you reach the dining room. Make one trip to the buffet line to prevent overeating. Try to get a cabin with a small refrigerator to store the snacks you need.

Useful References

Books

The Diabetes Travel Guide by Davida Kruger. Published by the American Diabetes Association, 2000.

American Diabetes Association Guide to Healthy Restaurant Eating by Hope Warshaw. Published by the American Diabetes Association, 2000.

Type 1 Diabetes

In type 1 diabetes, your body stops making insulin or makes only a small amount. When this happens, you must take insulin to stay healthy. Insulin is a hormone made in the pancreas. The pancreas releases insulin into the blood to help sugar from food get into body cells. If the body doesn't have enough insulin, the sugar cannot get into the cells. It stays in the blood and can make your blood glucose levels too high. After a number of years, diabetes can lead to serious problems in your eyes, kidneys, nerves, and blood vessels.

Type 1 diabetes occurs most often in childhood or the early teenage years. But it can occur at any age. The signs of type 1 diabetes can come on suddenly and be severe. The signs of type 1 diabetes are:

- Constant thirst (polydipsia)
- Frequent urination (polyuria)
- Constant hunger (polyphagia)
- Weakness and fatigue
- Weight loss

- Mood changes
- Nausea and vomiting

Type 1 diabetes is an autoimmune disease, which means that your body destroys its own cells. In type 1 diabetes the insulin-producing beta cells of the pancreas are destroyed. It is not clear why people develop type 1 diabetes. If you have a certain genetic makeup you may be more likely to get type 1 diabetes. Some believe there is an environmental trigger causing susceptible people to develop the disease.

The primary treatment goals for type 1 diabetes are to keep blood glucose levels as close to the normal range as possible. Treatment involves insulin, a healthy meal plan, regular exercise, and frequent blood glucose monitoring. People with type 1 diabetes take insulin injections or use an insulin pump.

The meal plan recommendations for people with type 1 diabetes focus on adjusting doses of insulin to the amount of carbohydrate intake and activity level. The meal plan should be designed to provide adequate calories for weight management goals. Several meal-planning approaches are available depending on your lifestyle and preferences.

Useful References

Web Sites

www.diabetes.org
www.niddk.nih.gov

Book

American Diabetes Association's Complete Guide to Diabetes, 2nd Edition. Published by the American Diabetes Association, 1999.

Type 2 Diabetes

Type 2 diabetes, formerly called adult-onset diabetes, is the most common form of the disease. In type 2 diabetes, your body does not make enough insulin or you may not be able to efficiently use the insulin you are making to turn the glucose in your blood into energy. The glucose remains in the bloodstream and reaches high levels, which can damage your eyes, nerves, heart, kidneys, and blood vessels.

Although most people diagnosed with type 2 diabetes are over 40 years of age, it has recently begun occurring more frequently in youth (see page 238). Symptoms of type 2 diabetes include:

- Constant thirst (polydipsia)
- Frequent urination (polyuria)
- Constant hunger (polyphagia)
- Weight loss
- Dry, itchy skin
- Tingling or numb hands or feet

- Fatigue or weakness
- Infections that recur or heal slowly
- Blurred vision

Type 2 diabetes can lead to a variety of problems with glucose metabolism: the pancreas doesn't produce enough insulin, the liver releases too much glucose, or the muscle cells don't readily take in glucose. Although researchers aren't sure of the exact cause of type 2 diabetes, they do know that a family history of type 2 diabetes and being overweight are key factors. Blood glucose monitoring, physical activity, and an individualized meal plan are important parts of treatment for type 2 diabetes. There are a variety of oral medications available to help control blood glucose (see page 183). It may be necessary to add insulin injections to the treatment plan.

While losing weight can improve your blood glucose if you have type 2 diabetes, your main goal should be to achieve the target levels of blood glucose, blood lipids, and blood pressure set by you and your diabetes team. An individualized nutrition plan with calories and carbohydrate spaced throughout the day, developed after an assessment by a registered dietitian, will start you in the right direction. Such a meal plan may involve a low fat, calorie-restricted diet with the correct amount of carbohydrate to control blood glucose.

Useful References

Web Sites

www.diabetes.org
www.niddk.nih.gov

Book

American Diabetes Association Complete Guide to Diabetes, 2nd Edition. Published by the American Diabetes Association, 1999.

Type 2 Diabetes in Youth

There has been growing concern about the recent sharp increase in reported cases of type 2 diabetes in children and adolescents. These children are usually overweight or obese when they are diagnosed. The signs and symptoms are similar to those of type 2 diabetes in adults.

The causes of type 2 diabetes in youth are unclear, but seem to be complex and relate to lifestyle, family history, and ethnicity. Puberty and the changes in hormone levels during this time cause insulin resistance and decreased insulin action. Obesity may be another factor that affects insulin resistance.

Treatment goals for type 2 diabetes in youth focus on keeping blood glucose levels in the normal range and decreasing the risk for other diseases such as high blood pressure and high blood lipid levels. This usually involves lifestyle modifications in diet and exercise, blood glucose monitoring, and eventually diabetes medications. Children with type 2 diabetes and their significant others should participate in a diabetes self-management course.

The goal of lifestyle interventions (exercise and meal planning) is to slow the rate of weight gain without affecting the child's growth. A low-fat meal plan approach for the whole family might be used. Regular physical activity will improve blood fat levels, decrease insulin resistance, and decrease body fat. Family involvement in lifestyle changes is essential for successful treatment.

Useful References

Web Sites

www.childrenwithdiabetes.com
www.diabetes.org

United Kingdom Prospective Diabetes Study (UKPDS)

The United Kingdom Prospective Diabetes Study (UKPDS) demonstrated that individuals with type 2 diabetes who were treated intensively over a period of 10 years had a 26% greater reduction in their risk of eye and kidney complications than those in a conventional treatment group. The study found that there was no difference between using insulin, sulfonylureas, or biguanides to achieve tight glucose control, although those using insulin tended to gain more weight than those using oral diabetes medicines. Intensive treatment also increased the risk of hypoglycemia.

The UKPDS also showed that lowering blood pressure to at least 144/82 mmHg in patients with type 2 diabetes reduced the incidence of strokes, diabetes-related deaths, heart failure, small vessel complications, and eye complications. Although this study began with a "diet only" group, almost 80% of the patients in the diet group had a medication added to their treatment plan when their fasting plasma glucose exceeded 270 mg/dl. The researchers noted that there is an increase in blood glucose levels with increased duration of type 2 diabetes, which may make medications necessary no matter how carefully a person with diabetes follows their meal plan.

The UKPDS proved that tight blood glucose control is beneficial in individuals with type 2 diabetes. This means that people with type 2 diabetes should take their condition seriously, rather than casually labeling it as "a touch of sugar." The results obtained in the UKPDS are possible for anyone with type 2 diabetes. See your diabetes team to intensify your efforts at diabetes control.

The Diabetes Control and Complications Trial (DCCT) demonstrated that intensive blood glucose control in patents with type 1 diabetes reduces the risk of developing eye disease, kidney disease, and nerve complications. (See page 64 for more information.)

Vegetarian Diets

Vegetarian diets can be a healthy choice for people with diabetes. Vegetarian diets are plant-based, meaning the majority of the foods eaten come from plants: fruits, vegetables, grains, beans, lentils, soybeans, nuts, and seeds. People become vegetarians for different reasons. Some people choose a vegetarian diet because of health reasons, environmental factors, food preferences, spiritual issues, or compassion for animals.

- **Lacto-ovo-vegetarians** choose a diet with eggs and dairy products, but no meat, poultry, seafood, and fish. "Lacto" refers to milk and "ovo" refers to eggs. Most vegetarians in the United States fit into this group.
- **Lacto-vegetarians** avoid meat, poultry, fish, seafood, and eggs, but not dairy products.
- **Vegans** avoid all foods of animal origin such as meat, poultry, fish, eggs, milk, cheese, and other dairy products. Vegans avoid all foods with animal products as ingredients.
- **Semi-vegetarians** mostly follow a vegetarian eating pattern but occasionally eat meat, poultry, or fish.

Eating vegetarian style offers advantages for good health. Vegetarians are less likely to be overweight, to have high cholesterol levels, or to have high blood pressure. Vegetarians are less likely to get heart disease and certain cancers. If you have type 1 diabetes, becoming vegetarian may enable you to use less insulin. If you switch to a vegetarian eating style with more fruits, vegetables, and grains, this may result in a higher carbohydrate intake. If you have type 2 diabetes, eating vegetarian style may help you lose weight. This will help with blood glucose control.

Being vegetarian doesn't necessarily mean that your diet is healthy or balanced. Like any way of eating, a vegetarian eating style can be high in fat and cholesterol. The nutritional content of a vegetarian diet depends on overall food choices. When properly planned, a vegetarian diet can provide all the essential nutrients needed for good health. If you are a vegetarian, ask your registered dietitian for helpful resources and meal planning tips to keep your diabetes under control and make sure you get all the nutrients you need. Try the tips below:

- Read vegetarian cookbooks for meal planning tips and recipes.
- Use the diabetes food guide pyramid to guide your food choices. Include the following foods every day:
    - 6 or more servings of grains, beans, and starchy vegetables
    - 3–5 servings of vegetables
    - 2–4 servings of fruit
    - 2–3 servings of milk or other calcium-rich food
    - 2–3 servings of protein foods such as legumes, tofu, eggs, cheese, or nuts
    - Fats, oils, alcohol, and sweets in moderation
- Stock up on vegetarian ingredients for quick cooking ideas.
- Make grain or bean dishes the centerpiece of your meal.

Useful References

- **Web Site**
  www.envirolink.org

- **Books**
  Being Vegetarian by Suzanne Havala. Published by John Wiley & Sons, 1998.

  Month of Meals: Vegetarian Pleasures by the American Diabetes Association, 1998.

Vitamins and Minerals

Most people with diabetes who eat a well-balanced diet do not require special vitamins and minerals. However, you may need a supplement if you fall into a high-risk group such as the elderly, pregnant or breastfeeding women, strict vegetarians, or those following a severely calorie-restricted diet. Several vitamins and minerals are of special interest if you have diabetes.

Antioxidant supplementation with **vitamins C, E, beta-carotene,** and **selenium** has been suggested, but long-term studies have failed to support those recommendations. There is also increasing interest in **folate** supplementation to lower elevated serum homocysteine levels and prevent heart disease, a common complication for people with diabetes. Research trials are still being conducted, but until the results are in you may want to boost your diet with naturally-occurring folate from foods such as leafy vegetables, legumes, and enriched grain products. The role of folate in preventing birth defects is widely accepted.

Nicotinamide is a form of Vitamin B3 that—when given in very large doses—may protect and improve the function of the beta cells in the pancreas. A large-scale research study is currently being conducted to determine if nicotinamide can prevent type 1 diabetes in children. Until the results are in, you should avoid large supplements of nicotinamide because of potential side effects such as headache and skin reactions, as well as gastrointestinal and liver problems.

Chromium, magnesium, and vanadium are the minerals most commonly mentioned as potential supplements for people with diabetes. **Chromium** is a trace element that works with insulin to help the body use glucose more effectively. Several studies have shown positive effects of chromium supplementation on diabetes control, particularly if an individual is chromium-deficient. However, there is not enough evidence to recommend chromium supplementation for all people with diabetes. Chromium supplements can have dangerous side effects, including kidney failure, liver problems, and severe low blood glucose (hypoglycemia). Chromium is found in food sources such as Brewers yeast, oysters, mushrooms, liver, potatoes, beef, cheese, and fresh vegetables.

Magnesium is one of the few minerals that is commonly deficient in people with diabetes, although it is difficult to determine magnesium status in the body. Magnesium assists in transporting glucose in the body, and a relationship has been shown between low magnesium intake and insulin resistance in people without diabetes. People at high risk for magnesium deficiency who may benefit from supplementation include those with congestive heart failure or acute myocardial infarction, ketoacidosis, alcohol abuse problems, long-term parenteral nutrition needs, calcium or potassium deficiency, chronic use of certain drugs, and pregnant women. Good food sources of magnesium are whole grains, dark green leafy vegetables, nuts, legumes, and fish.

Vanadium is a trace element found in several foods including grains, sunflower seeds, vegetables, wine, and beer. Although it may increase the body's sensitivity to insulin, the only scientific studies of vanadium are very small scale. Vanadium can cause gastrointestinal side effects, accumulate in body tissues, and is potentially quite toxic. Vanadium supplementation is not recommended at this time.

Although vitamin and minerals are "natural" substances, they can have serious side effects. If you are interested in supplementing your meal plan with a vitamin or mineral, talk with your diabetes team and follow the guidelines for safe supplement use. (See page 136 for more information.)

Weight Control

Losing weight is one of the single greatest steps people with type 2 diabetes can take to bring their diabetes under control. Losing weight will lower blood pressure, lower the risk for heart disease, and improve blood glucose control. It is common for people with type 2 diabetes who are initially prescribed insulin or oral diabetes medicines to find that once they lose weight they can control their diabetes with diet alone.

Having too much fat, especially on the upper body (apple-shaped body), decreases the body's ability to use insulin. This is called insulin resistance. Weight loss lowers insulin resistance. This allows your natural insulin (in people with type 2 diabetes) to do a better job lowering blood glucose levels.

Weight control improves blood fat and blood pressure levels. People with diabetes are about twice as likely to get cardiovascular disease as most people. Lowering blood fats and blood pressure is a way to reduce that risk.

If you are overweight, check with your health care professionals about how much weight loss would be good for you. Make your health, not your appearance, your weight management priority. The best approach to weight loss is a combination of exercise and a healthy diet. No one plan works for everyone. Some people find it easier to restrict their calories, while other find it easier to increase their activity. Usually a combination of both is the most successful. Whatever strategy you choose, decide that the changes you make will be a lifetime plan that requires some new ways of thinking instead of a brief episode in your life. Permanent changes keep the weight off.

Many meal plan approaches are available for weight control. Discuss your weight loss goals and meal plan options with your registered dietitian and select the approach that fits your lifestyle. A repeated cycle of weight loss and weight gain isn't the best approach to weight management. The calorie level should allow a slow gradual weight loss over several months. These diet and eating tips will get you started:

- Cut back on fat in your food choices.
- Include more fruits, vegetables, and whole grains.
- Control your portions.
- Choose snacks wisely.
- Avoid skipping meals.
- Plan your meals and snacks ahead of time.
- Portion food before you bring it to the table.
- Eat slowly and sit down to eat.
- Learn your triggers for overeating.
- Celebrate your successes.

Your plan should include increased physical activity, daily or several times a week. Keep variety, balance, and moderation in mind when you plan your exercise. Enjoy different activities that exercise different muscles, including your heart. To achieve overall fitness, include exercises that build cardiovascular endurance, muscular strength, bone strength, and flexibility. Exercise to keep fit with 30 minutes or more of moderate exercise in your daily routine, most days of the week.

Useful References

- **Web Sites**
  www.niddk.nih.gov
  www.caloriecontrol.org

- **Books**
  The Commonsense Guide to Weight Loss for People with Diabetes by Barbara Caleen Hansen and Shauna S. Roberts. Published by the American Diabetes Association, 1998.

  The Complete Weight Loss Workbook by Judith Wylie-Rosett, ed. Published by the American Diabetes Association, 1998.

Whole Grains

When grains are milled, or refined, the bran and germ portions are removed, leaving only the endosperm. Unlike refined grains, whole grains include all the healthy parts of a grain: the bran, endosperm, and the germ. These components provide nutrients and food components that benefit health. Consumption of whole grains has been linked to reduced risk for heart disease, diabetes, and certain cancers. Antioxidants and dietary fiber contained in whole grains may lower cholesterol and lower the risk for heart disease.

Eating whole-grain foods may decrease the risk of developing type 2 diabetes. In people with diabetes, whole grains appear to influence carbohydrate metabolism and improve glycemic control. Recent research indicates that whole grain consumption improves glycemic control, decreases insulin resistance, and decreases fasting insulin levels.

Wheat, corn, oats, and rice are the most common varieties of grain eaten in the United States. Many foods are made from these grains: breads, cereals, pasta, and crackers. The phrase "whole grain" tells you that the food is made from the entire grain. To find foods that have

Whole-Grain Food	One Serving
Cereals	3/4 cup to 1 cup ready-to-eat cereal
	1/2 cup cooked cereal
Breads	1 slice bread
	1 small roll
	1/2 bagel
	1/2 hamburger bun
Brown rice	1/2 cup cooked
Pasta	1/2 cup cooked
Pancakes	2 small
Waffles	1 small
Muffins	1 small
Crackers	3 or 4 small

whole grains, read both the ingredient list and the Nutrition Facts panel. Pick foods that contain two or more grams of dietary fiber. Look for foods with these ingredients listed first on the ingredient listing:

- Whole-grain oats
- Whole-grain wheat or whole wheat
- Whole-grain barley
- Whole-grain corn

Good food sources of whole grain are also able to list the health claim that they may reduce the risk of heart disease and certain cancers. Ask your registered dietitian for help in increasing your intake of whole-grain foods.

Index

A

Acesulfame K, 117, 198, 224
Acupuncture, 175
Adequate intake (AI), 71–72
Adolescence, 1–2
Adult-onset diabetes. *see* Type 2 diabetes
Aerobic exercise, 89, 91–92
Air travel, 232–233
Alcohol, 3–4
  ADA guidelines, 180
  food pyramid, 68
  high blood pressure and, 145
  during pregnancy, 117, 198
Alpha-glucosidase inhibitors, 184
Alternative therapies, 175
American Association of Diabetes Educators (AADE), 5
American Diabetes Association (ADA), 6
  cookbooks, 205
  nutrition guidelines, 178–180
American Dietetic Association (ADA), 7
  cookbooks, 205
Angina, 133
Anorexia nervosa, 75–76
Antioxidants, 8–9, 245
Appetite suppressants, 10–11
Artificial sweeteners. *see* Sugar substitutes
Aspartame, 117, 198, 224
Athletes, 12–13. *see also* Exercise
  carbohydrate loading, 37–38
  electrolytes, 82–83
Automobile, travel by, 232

B

Basal calories, 29
Beans, 66–68, 164–165
Behavior change, stages of, 14–15
Beta-carotene, 8–9, 245
Biguanides, 185
Birth defects, 196
Blood glucose control
  blood fat levels and, 17
  breastfeeding and, 25–26
  carbohydrate counting, 34–36
  for children aged 6–11, 45
  during exercise, 89–90
  during pregnancy, 115–116

Blood glucose levels, 20–21
  alcohol and, 3–4
  caffeine and, 27–28
  carbohydrates and, 31–33
  dawn phenomenon, 141–142
  dietary supplements to lower, 136–137
  eating disorders and, 75–76
  exercise and, 12–13, 88–90
  high. *see* Hyperglycemia
  low. *see* Hypoglycemia
  metabolism and, 172–173
  during pregnancy, 196–197
  Somogyi effect, 142
Blood glucose monitoring, 22–24
  after exercise, 92
  breastfeeding and, 25–26
  dietary supplements and, 138
  during exercise, 89–90
  fructosamine test, 113–114
  glycohemoglobin test, 124–125
  goal guidelines, 23
  during honeymoon phase, 139
  patterns, finding, 23–24
Blood lipids (fats), 16–19
Body mass index (BMI), 182
Bowel health
  constipation, 52–53
  diverticulosis, 73–74
Breastfeeding, 25–26
  advantages of, 58–59
  caffeine and, 28
  calorie adjustments for, 30
  cow's milk *vs.*, 58–59
Bulimia, 75–76

C
Caffeine, 27–28
  during pregnancy, 117, 198
Calcium, 80–81
  ADA guidelines, 179–180
  osteoporosis and, 186–188
  sources of, 187–188
Calorie point system, 191
Calories, 29–30
  burned in various activities, 91–92
  pregnancy requirements, 197
Carbohydrate-based fat replacers, 95
Carbohydrate counting, 34–36
  choice method, 192
  fiber adjustments, 102, 165
  gram, defined, 128
  insulin pumps and, 153
Carbohydrate loading, 37–38
Carbohydrates, 31–33
  ADA guidelines, 179
  exchange list, 86
  exercise and, 12–13
  fiber. *see* Fiber
  grams of, on food labels, 108
  sugars/sweets, 31–32, 68, 226–227
  whole grains, 251–252
Carbohydrate-to-insulin ratio, 39–40
Celiac disease, 41–42
Certified diabetes educators (CDEs), 5, 43–44, 208
Cheese, 67–68, 188

Chest pain (angina), 133
Children
  herbal supplements and, 137
  6-11 years old, 45–46
  teens, 1–2
  toddlers, 228–229
  type 2 diabetes in, 238–239
Chloride, 82–83
Cholesterol
  dietary, 47–48, 78–79
    ADA guidelines, 179
    exercise reducing, 88
  serum (blood), 16–18
Chromium, 246
Complementary therapies, 175
Complications, 49–51
  eye disease, 50–51
  intensive therapy and, 64–65, 240–241
  kidney disease. *see* Kidney disease
Constipation, 52–53
Convenience foods, 54–55
Conventional diabetes therapy, 56–57
Cookbooks, 205–206
Cornstarch, 209
Cow's milk, 58–59, 67–68
Cruises, 233

D

Dairy products, 67–68. *see also* Milk
  calcium in, 187–188
DASH diet, 60–61, 145
Dawn phenomenon, 141–142
Dehydration, 62–63
  caffeine and, 28
  electrolyte depletion, 82–83
  exercise and, 91
Desirable body weight, 181–182
Diabetes Control and Complications Trial (DCCT), 64–65
Diabetes food pyramid, 66–68, 103–104
Diabetes management
  alternative therapies, 175
  behavior change, stages of, 14–15
  blood glucose monitoring. *see* Blood glucose monitoring
  conventional therapy, 56–57
  for the elderly, 80–81
  goal setting, 126–127
  honeymoon phase, 139–140
  insulin pump therapy, 152–153
  intensive therapy, 64–65, 240–241
  ketones, 159–160
  meal planning. *see* Meal planning
  on special occasions, 220–221
Diabetes Prevention Program (DPP), 201
Diabetes Prevention Trial—Type 1 (DPT—1), 201
Diabetic ketoacidosis (DKA), 141, 160
Dialysis, 161–162
Dietary Guidelines for Americans, 69–70

Dietary reference intakes (DRIs), 71–72
Dietary supplements, 136–138, 175, 245–247
  ADA guidelines, 179–180
  antioxidants, 8–9, 245
  calcium, 80–81, 179–180, 188
  dietary reference intakes (DRIs), 71–72
  for the elderly, 80–81
  fish oil, 98
  phytochemicals, 177
  prenatal, 117, 197–198
  safe use of, 137–138
Diet pills, 10–11
Diverticulosis, 73–74
D-phenylalanine derivative, 184
Dry beans, 67–68

E

Eating disorders, 75–77
Eggs, 67–68, 78–79
Elderly, 80–81
  diverticulosis, 73–74
Electrolytes, 82–83
Estimated average requirement (EAR), 72
Estrogen replacement therapy, 187
Ethnic foods, 84–85
Exchange lists, 86–87
  alcoholic beverages, 4
  legumes, 165
Exchange Lists for Meal Planning, 86–87
Exercise, 88–92
  athletes. *see* Athletes
  benefits of, 88
  blood fat levels and, 18
  blood glucose levels, maintaining, 89–90
  complications and, 50
  fluid intake during, 63, 82, 91
  ketone levels and, 89
  snacks and, 89, 90
  timing of workouts, 89
  vacations/holidays and, 220
  weight control and, 249–250
Eye disease, 50–51

F

Fast food, 93–94
Fat-based fat replacers, 96
Fat counting approach, 192
Fat replacers, 95–96
Fats, 97–100
  ADA guidelines, 179
  blood lipids, 16–19
  cholesterol. *see* Cholesterol
  diabetes risk, reducing, 201
  exchange list, 87
  food pyramid, 68
  grams of, on food labels, 108
  lowering intake of, 99–100
  monounsaturated, 18, 97, 99
  polyunsaturated, 97–98, 99
  replacements for, 95–96
  saturated, 18, 98, 99
Fiber, 31–32, 101–102
  ADA guidelines, 179
  cholesterol and, 18
  constipation, preventing, 52–53
  diabetes risk, reducing, 202

diverticulosis and, 73–74
legumes, 164–165
The First Step in Diabetes Meal Planning, 103–104
Fish, 67–68
omega-3 fatty acids, 98, 99
during pregnancy, 117, 198
Fluid requirements, 62–63
constipation, preventing, 52
electrolytes and, 82–83
during exercise, 91
renal diet and, 163
Folate, 245
Food diaries, 105–106
Food labels, 107–108, 130
percent daily values, 189–190
Food safety, 109–110
eggs, 79
during pregnancy, 117, 198
Foot care, 50
Free foods, 111–112
Fructosamine test, 113–114
Fructose, 227
Fruit group, food pyramid, 67–68
Functional foods, 176

G

Gestational diabetes mellitus (GDM), 115–117. *see also* Pregnancy
Glucagon, 118–119
Glucose intolerance, 120–121
Gluten, 41–42
Glycemic index, 122–123
Glycohemoglobin test, 124–125
Goal setting, 126–127
Grains, food pyramid, 66–68
Gram, 128
Grocery shopping, 129–130

H

Health claims, on food labels, 108
Healthy Food Choices, 131–132
Heart attack, 133. *see also* Heart disease
Heart disease, 133–135
exercise and, 88
glucose intolerance and, 120–121
saturated fats and, 98
Herbals, 136–138
High blood pressure, 49–50, 144–145
DASH diet for, 60–61
diabetes complications and, 240–241
exercise reducing, 88
potassium supplements, 83
High-density lipoproteins (HDLs), 17
High-protein diets, 166–167
Holidays, 220–221
Honeymoon phase, 139–140
Hyperglycemia, 20, 141–143
Somogyi effect, 142
Hyperglycemic hyperosmolar nonketotic syndrome (HHNS), 142
Hypertension. *see* High blood pressure
Hypoglycemia, 21, 146–148
delayed, after exercise, 92

Hypoglycemia (*continued*)
eating disorders and, 76
glucagon injections for, 118–119
oral diabetes medications and, 183–185
resistant starch and, 209
severe, treatment of, 118–119
in toddlers, 228

I

Illness, 212–213
dehydration and, 63, 82–83, 212
foodborne, 109–110
ketones and, 159–160, 212
Impaired fasting glucose (IFG), 120
Impaired glucose tolerance (IGT), 120
Infant formula, 58–59
Ingredient list, on food labels, 107
Insulin, 149–151
carbohydrate-to-insulin ratio, 39–40
conventional therapy, 56–57
exercise and, 12–13
oral, development of, 185
storage tips, 150–151
toddlers, dosing for, 228–229
types of, 149–150
Insulin pumps, 152–153
Insulin reaction. *see* Hypoglycemia
Insulin resistance, 120–121
Insurance, medical nutrition therapy coverage, 171
Intensive diabetes therapy, 64–65, 154–156, 240–241
hypoglycemic unawareness, 146
Internet, 157–158

K

Ketones, 159–160
exercise and, 89
Kidney disease, 161–163
protein intake and, 203
salt substitutes and, 217

L

Lacto-ovo-vegetarians, 242
Lacto-vegetarians, 242
Laxatives, 53
Legumes, 164–165
Lipoproteins, 16–17
Low-carbohydrate diets, 166–167
Low-density lipoproteins (LDLs), 17

M

Magnesium, 246
Meal planning, 168–169
ADA nutrition guidelines, 178–180
carbohydrate counting approach, 34–36
for children aged 6-11, 45–46
complications and, 50
convenience foods, 54–55
DASH diet, 60–61

diabetes food pyramid, 66–68, 103–104
Dietary Guidelines for Americans, 69–70
for the elderly, 80–81
ethnic foods, 84–85
Exchange Lists for Meal Planning, 86–87
fast food, 93–94
The First Step in Diabetes Meal Planning, 103–104
food diaries, 105–106
food label information, 107–108
free foods, 111–112
glycemic index, 122–123
grocery shopping tips, 129–130
Healthy Food Choices, 131–132
during honeymoon phase, 139
intensive therapy and, 65, 155
legumes, 164–165
point systems, 191–193
portion control, 194–195
during pregnancy, 116–117, 197–198
registered dietitians and, 207–208
renal diet, 162–163
snacks. *see* Snacks
total available glucose (TAG) approach, 230
vegetarian diets, 242–244
Meat
cholesterol content of, 48
exchange list, 86
food pyramid, 67–68
Medical foods, 170
Medical nutrition therapy (MNT), 171
Medicare, medical nutrition therapy coverage, 171
Meglitinides, 184
Metabolism, 172–173
Milk, 58–59
food pyramid, 67–68
soy, 219
Minerals, 245–247. *see also* Dietary supplements
ADA guidelines, 179–180
pregnancy needs, 197–198
Miscarriage, 196
Monounsaturated fats, 18, 97, 99
Month of Meals, 169

N

National Certification Board for Diabetes Educators (NCBDE), 43, 44
National Diabetes Education Program (NDEP), 174
National Digestive Disease Information Clearinghouse, 74
National Institute of Diabetes, Digestive, and Kidney Disease (NIDDK), 74
Nephropathy. *see* Kidney disease
Nerve disease (neuropathy), 51, 175
Nicotinamide, 245–246

Nutrition
  ADA guidelines, 178–180
  alternative/complementary therapies, 175
  dietary reference intakes (DRIs), 71–72
  food label information, 107–108
  functional foods, 176
  organic foods, 176
  phytochemicals, 176–177
Nuts, 67–68

O

Obesity, 181–182
  appetite suppressants, 10–11
  type 2 diabetes in youth, 238–239
Oils. *see* Fats
Omega-3 fatty acids, 98, 99
Oral diabetes medications, 183–185
Organic foods, 176
Osteoporosis, 186–188

P

Parties, 221
Peanuts, 164–165
Percent daily values (%DV), 189–190
Peripheral vascular disease, 134
Phosphorus, 163
Physical activity. *see* Exercise
Phytochemicals, 176–177
Plasma glucose levels, 23
Plus activity calories, 29
Point systems, 191–193
Polycystic ovary disease, 121
Polyols (sugar alcohols), 222–223
Polyunsaturated fats, 97–98, 99
Portion control, 194–195
Potassium, 82–83, 163
Poultry, 67–68
Pregnancy, 196–199
  blood glucose goals, 115–116, 196–197
  blood glucose monitoring and, 22, 115
  breastfeeding, 25–26
  caffeine and, 28, 117, 198
  calorie adjustments for, 30, 197
  dietary supplements and, 137
  fish, warnings about, 117, 198
  fructosamine testing, 113–114
  gestational diabetes, 115–117
  hypoglycemic unawareness, 146
  ketones and, 159–160
  nutritional goals, 116–117, 197–198
  weight gain, 116, 197
Prevention of diabetes, 200–202
Protein, 203–204
  ADA guidelines, 179
  renal diet and, 163
  soy products, 218–219
Protein-based fat replacers, 95–96

R

Raw fish, 117, 198
Recipes, 205–206

Recommended dietary allowance (RDA), 71
Record-keeping
carbohydrate-to-insulin ratio, 39
patterns, finding, 23–24
Registered dietitians (RDs), 7, 207–208
meal planning, 168–169
medical nutrition therapy, 171
Renal diet, 162–163
Resistant starch, 209
Restaurant dining, 210–211
Retinopathy, 50–51

S
Saccharin, 117, 198, 224
Safe handling. *see* Food safety
Salt. *see* Sodium
Salt substitutes, 217
Saturated fats, 18, 98, 99
Selenium, 8–9, 245
Semi-vegetarians, 242
Serving size, on food labels, 108
Sick days. *see* Illness
Smoking, 18, 50
Snacks, 214–215
breastfeeding and, 26
for children aged 6–11, 46
during exercise, 89, 90
medical snack bars, 170
when traveling, 232
Sodium, 82–83, 216–217
ADA guidelines, 179
high blood pressure and, 144–145
Somogyi effect, 142
Soybeans, 164–165
Soy products, 218–219
Special occasions, 220–221
Starches, 31–32, 66–68, 209
Stroke, 134
saturated fats and, 98
Sucralose, 117, 198, 225
Sugar alcohols, 222–223
Sugars/Sweets, 31–32, 68, 226–227
Sugar substitutes, 224–225
during pregnancy, 117, 198
sugar alcohols, 222–223
Sulfonylurea/Biguanide, 184
Sulfonylureas, 183
Syndrome X, 120–121

T
Table salt, 216
Teenagers, 1–2
Tempeh, 219
Textured soy protein, 219
Thiazolidinediones, 184
Tight control. *see* Intensive diabetes therapy
Toddlers, 228–229
Tofu, 219
Tolerable upper intake level (UL), 72
Total available glucose (TAG), 230
Trans fatty acids, 18, 98–99
Travel, 231–233
Triglycerides, 16–18

Type 1 diabetes, 234–235
  blood glucose monitoring and, 22
  celiac disease and, 41–42
  conventional therapy, 56–57
  cow's milk and development of, 58–59
  honeymoon phase, 139–140
  intensive therapy for, 154–156
  prevention, 200–202
  risk factors, 200
  symptoms, 234–235
Type 2 diabetes, 236–239
  blood fat levels and, 17
  blood glucose monitoring and, 23
  complications, preventing, 65
  exercise, benefits of, 88
  glucose intolerance and, 120–121
  high-fiber diet and, 101
  hyperglycemic hyperosmolar nonketotic syndrome (HHNS), 142
  intensive therapy for, 154–156, 240–241
  oral medications, 183–185
  prevention, 200–202
  risk factors, 200–201
  snacks and, 214
  symptoms, 236–237
  United Kingdom Prospective Diabetes Study (UKPDS), 65, 240–241
  weight control, importance of, 248
  Weight Watchers 1-2-3 Success Point System, 192
  in youth, 238–239

U

United Kingdom Prospective Diabetes Study (UKPDS), 65, 240–241

V

Vanadium, 246–247
Vegans, 242
Vegetable group, food pyramid, 67–68
Vegetarian diets, 242–244
Very-low-density lipoproteins (VLDLs), 16
Vitamin A, 8–9, 245
Vitamin C, 8–9, 245
Vitamin D, 187
Vitamin E, 8–9, 245
Vitamins, 245–247. *see also* Dietary supplements
  ADA guidelines, 179–180
  pregnancy needs, 197–198

W

Waist-to-hip ratio, 182
Web sites, nutrition, 157–158
Weight control, 181–182, 248–250
  appetite suppressants, 10–11
  blood fats and, 18
  body mass index (BMI), 182
  calorie adjustments for, 30
  calories burned by various activities, 91–92

desirable body weight, 181–182
diabetes risk and, 201
high blood pressure and, 144
low-carbohydrate/high protein diets, 166–167
during pregnancy, 116, 197
waist-to-hip ratio, 182
Weight Watchers 1-2-3 Success Point System, 192
Whole grains, 251–252

Y

Yogurt, 67–68, 188

About the American Diabetes Association

The American Diabetes Association is the nation's leading voluntary health organization supporting diabetes research, information, and advocacy. Its mission is to prevent and cure diabetes and to improve the lives of all people affected by diabetes. The American Diabetes Association is the leading publisher of comprehensive diabetes information. Its huge library of practical and authoritative books for people with diabetes covers every aspect of self-care—cooking and nutrition, fitness, weight control, medications, complications, emotional issues, and general self-care.

To order American Diabetes Association books: Call 1-800-232-6733. http://store.diabetes.org (Note: there is no need to use **www** when typing this particular Web address.)

To join the American Diabetes Association: Call 1-800-806-7801. www.diabetes.org/membership

For more information about diabetes or ADA programs and services: Call 1-800-342-2383. E-mail: Customerservice@diabetes.org

To locate an ADA/NCQA Recognized Provider of quality diabetes care in your area: Call 1-703-549-1500 ext. 2202. www.diabetes.org/recognition/Physicians/ListAll.asp

To find an ADA Recognized Education Program in your area: Call 1-888-232-0822. www.diabetes.org/recognition/education.asp

To join the fight to increase funding for diabetes research, end discrimination, and improve insurance coverage: Call 1-800-342-2383. www.diabetes.org/advocacy

To find out how you can get involved with the programs in your community: Call 1-800-342-2383. See below for program Web addresses.

- *American Diabetes Month:* Educational activities aimed at those diagnosed with diabetes—month of November. www.diabetes.org/ADM
- *American Diabetes Alert:* Annual public awareness campaign to find the undiagnosed—held the fourth Tuesday in March. www.diabetes.org/alert
- *The Diabetes Assistance & Resources Program (DAR):* diabetes awareness program targeted to the Latino community. www.diabetes.org/DAR
- *African American Program:* diabetes awareness program targeted to the African American community. www.diabetes.org/africanamerican
- *Awakening the Spirit: Pathways to Diabetes Prevention & Control:* diabetes awareness program targeted to the Native American community. www.diabetes.org/awakening

To find out about an important research project regarding type 2 diabetes: www.diabetes.org/ada/research.asp

To obtain information on making a planned gift or charitable bequest: Call 1-888-700-7029. www.diabetes.org/ada/plan.asp

To make a donation or memorial contribution: Call 1-800-342-2383. www.diabetes.org/ada/cont.asp